Assisted Reproductive Technologies and Infectious Diseases

Andrea Borini • Valeria Savasi
Editors

Assisted Reproductive Technologies and Infectious Diseases

A Guide to Management

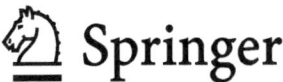 Springer

Editors
Andrea Borini, MD
Scientific Director
9.baby
Center for Fertility and Family
  Health
Bologna, Italy

Valeria Savasi, MD, PhD
Chief of Reproductive Unit
Unit of Obstetrics and
  Gynecology
Department of Biomedical
  and Clinical Sciences
Hospital "L. Sacco"
University of Milan
Milan, Italy

ISBN 978-3-319-30110-5   ISBN 978-3-319-30112-9   (eBook)
DOI 10.1007/978-3-319-30112-9

Library of Congress Control Number: 2016943072

Printed on acid-free paper

This Springer imprint is published by Springer Nature
The registered company is Springer International Publishing AG Switzerland

Preface

The idea of a book focusing on the infectious diseases and assisted reproductive technologies (ART) was born 3 years ago because reproductive assistance in subjects infected with blood viruses is still a complex issue. When we sat down to plan the first edition of this book, we were determined to make it innovative, comprehensive and accessible. We contacted the most important researchers in infectious diseases and ART in the world, and we asked them if they would be interested in participating in this project.

The infectious diseases involved in ART are various, but we decided to concentrate our attention on only some of them, and we chose the viral infections. Viral infections are the most interesting infections because the viruses are changeable, unpredictable, and most are untreatable. The word *virus* has a much longer history than the study of what we now call by that name. It comes directly from the Latin *virus*, a term meaning, "poison, sap of plants, slimy liquid". Its earliest known use in English to denote a disease-causing agent was in 1728, although for the rest of the eighteenth century, throughout the nineteenth and for several decades beyond, there was no clear distinction between virus as a vague term, applicable to any infectious microbe, and the very particular group of entities we know as viruses today. Moreover, some viruses create chronic infectious diseases: the most important are human immunodeficiency virus-1 (HIV-1), hepatitis C virus (HCV) and hepatitis B virus (HBV) infections. All of these chronic infections are ubiquitous and very dangerous because each of these viruses can lead to a widespread outbreak. Some outbreaks of viral disease quickly escalate, depending on viral transmissibility and virulence. These are the crucial parameters. For the blood-borne viruses, transmission is more complicated than for other types of virus. Generally, it depends on a third party: a vector. The viruses have to replicate in the blood of the host to produce severe viraemia. The vector—an insect, for example—must arrive for a meal, bite the host, slurp up the virions along with the blood, and carry them away. The yellow fever virus transmits this way. However, blood-borne viruses can also spread to new hosts by way of needles. Ebola, HIV and HCV, three viruses of very different characters and very different adaptive strategies, all happen to move well via needles. Sexual transmission is a good scheme for viruses with a low degree of hardiness in the external environment. Transmission during coitus is a conservative strategy, avoiding the risk of air or sun contact. Whatever the case, the sexually transmitted viruses tend towards patience. They cause persistent infections and endure long periods of latency (e.g. the herpes virus), or they replicate slowly (as with HIV and HBV).

In the last few years, clinicians have learned to treat an HIV infection with drugs, an HBV infection with a vaccine, an HVC infection with some drugs, and this situation has opened the door for the patient's desire to have children. Even in the presence of a chronic infection, or probably because the infection is chronic and well controlled, people need to have progeny. For this reason, clinicians have to address the patient's requests regarding pregnancies, and they have to try to save pregnancies and newborn babies. HBV infection seems to have minor relevance because a vaccine is available, but in the very near future the HBV virus will be able to change; if that happens, clinicians will be able to assist their infected patients. For the HIV virus, we have to consider that three quarters of individuals infected with it are in their reproductive years and may consider pregnancy planning. Techniques have been developed that can minimise the risk of HIV transmission in these couples, and ART programmes should be integrated into global public health services against HIV.

Regarding the HCV virus, the debate on HCV-discordant couples requiring ART is still open. Sexual transmission of HCV is a controversial issue, whereas the presence of the virus in the sperm has already been demonstrated. In ART, HCV transmission raises some questions. One of these is that specific guidelines regarding the behaviour of physicians in reproductive medicine have not yet been established. Thus, this book will try to answer many of the questions about these issues, obtaining a picture of the biological aspects of HIV, HCV and HBV infections and the real data presented in the literature regarding reproductive aspects in their presence. Finally, there is a chapter discussing the reproductive possibilities in poorer countries in Africa and South America, where these infectious diseases are more prevalent.

It is our hope that this resource will be of assistance to physicians and scientists engaged in this exciting field of medicine.

Bologna, Italy   Andrea Borini
Milan, Italy   Valeria Savasi

Contents

Contributors

Irene Cetin, MD Unit of Obstetrics and Gynecology, Department of Mother and Child, Luigi Sacco, Milan, Italy

Massimo Ciccozzi, MD, PhD Dipartimento Malattie Infettive, Parassitarie ed Immunomediate, Istituto Superiore di Sanità, Rome, Italy

Oriol Coll, MD, PhD Clinica Eugin, Barcelona, Spain

Fabienne Devreker, MD, PhD Laboratory for Research in Human Reproduction, Medicine Faculty, Department of Obstetrics and Gynecology, Hôpital Erasme, Université Libre de Bruxelles (ULB), Brussels, Belgium

Erika Ebranati, PhD Dipartimento di Scienze Cliniche e Biomediche "Luigi Sacco", Sezione di Malattie Infettive, Università degli Studi di Milano, Milan, Italy

Rocio Rivera, MSc Andrology Laboratory, Instituto Universitario IVI Valencia, Valencia, Spain

Yvon Englert, MD, PhD, MBA Laboratory for Research in Human Reproduction, Medicine Faculty, Department of Obstetrics and Gynecology, Hôpital Erasme, Université Libre de Bruxelles (ULB), Brussels, Belgium

Mᵃ Carmen Galbis, PhD, MSc Andrology Laboratory, Instituto Universitario IVI Valencia, Valencia, Spain

Ophthalmology Investigation, Hospital Universitario Dr. Peset, Valencia, Spain

Lisa Fiaschi Dipartimento di Scienze Cliniche e Biomediche "Luigi Sacco", Sezione di Malattie Infettive, Università degli Studi di Milano, Milan, Italy

Massimo Galli Dipartimento di Scienze Cliniche e Biomediche "Luigi Sacco", Sezione di Malattie Infettive, Università degli Studi di Milano, Milan, Italy

Xiao-Ling Hu, PhD Department of Reproductive Endocrinology, Women's Hospital, School of Medicine, Zhejiang University, Hangzhou, China

Arianna Laoreti, MD Unit of Obstetrics and Gynecology, Department of Mother and Child, Luigi Sacco, Milan, Italy

Elisabeth van Leeuwen, MD, PhD Department of Obstetrics and Gynecology, Academic Medical Center, Amsterdam, The Netherlands

Miao Li, MD Department of Reproductive Endocrinology, Women's Hospital, School of Medicine, Zhejiang University, Hangzhou, China

Luca Mandia, MD Department of Gynecology and Obstetrics, University of Milan, Milan, Italy

Daniel Mataró, MD, PhD Clinica Eugin, Barcelona, Spain

Hui-Hui Pan Department of Reproductive Endocrinology, Women's Hospital, School of Medicine, Zhejiang University, Hangzhou, China

Nicolás Garrido Puchalt, PhD, MSc Andrology Laboratory, Instituto Universitario IVI Valencia, Valencia, Spain

Asma Sassi, MD Laboratory for Research in Human Reproduction, Medicine Faculty, Department of Obstetrics and Gynecology, Hôpital Erasme, Université Libre de Bruxelles (ULB), Brussels, Belgium

Valeria Savasi, MD, PhD Unit of Obstetrics and Gynecology, Department of Biomedical and Clinical Sciences, Hospital "L. Sacco", University of Milan, Milan, Italy

Rita Vassena, DVM, PhD Clinica Eugin, Barcelona, Spain

Valérie Vernaeve, MD, PhD Clinica Eugin, Barcelona, Spain

Jia-Li You, MD Department of Reproductive Endocrinology, Women's Hospital, School of Medicine, Zhejiang University, Hangzhou, China

Valley Medical Oncology Consultants, Mountain View, CA, USA

Gianguglielmo   Zehender,   PhD Dipartimento   di   Scienze Cliniche e Biomediche "Luigi Sacco", Sezione di Malattie Infettive, Università degli Studi di Milano, Milan, Italy

Yi-Min Zhu, PhD Department of Reproductive Endocrinology, Women's Hospital, School of Medicine, Zhejiang University, Hangzhou, China

Chapter 1
The Impact of Human Immunodeficiency Virus (HIV) and Hepatitis B Virus (HBV) and Hepatitis C Virus (HCV) on Male and Female Fertility

Elisabeth van Leeuwen

Introduction

Every year, men and women infected with human immunodeficiency virus (HIV), hepatitis B (HBV) and hepatitis C (HCV) alone or with a combination of any of these infections consult their physician or gynaecologist because they are considering having offspring. Often, they have questions about whether the infection they have or the medication they are taking to control the infection is affecting their fertility status.

Couples living with HIV, HBV or HCV may have an increased need for assisted reproductive techniques (ART) to prevent transmission of the virus, and fertility screening has identified a high incidence of male and tubal factor subfertility among couples living with HIV, HBV and/or HCV [1].

The risk of sexual transmission is different for the three viruses. For HIV and HCV the main goal of treatment is often to reduce the transmission risks, but for HBV it is infertility treatment, as sexual

E. van Leeuwen, MD, PhD (✉)
Department of Obstetrics and Gynecology, Academic Medical Center,
Meibergdreef 9, Room H4-274, Amsterdam 1105 AZ, The Netherlands
e-mail: e.vanleeuwen@amc.nl

© Springer International Publishing Switzerland 2016   1
A. Borini, V. Savasi (eds.), *Assisted Reproductive
Technologies and Infectious Diseases*,
DOI 10.1007/978-3-319-30112-9_1

Table 1.1 Indications for assisted reproductive techniques (ART)

	HIV	HBV	HCV
Man negative Woman positive	Subfertility	Subfertility	Subfertility
Man positive Woman negative	Prevent transmission Subfertility	Subfertility	Prevent transmission Subfertility
Both partners infected	Subfertility, indication for ART when there is a risk of superinfection with resistant virus	Subfertility	Subfertility

partners can be vaccinated against HBV. Table 1.1 displays the different primary indications for ART for the different types of viral infections. Figure 1.1 displays the possible transmission of viruses in ART. Horizontal transmission is infection of a partner, vertical transmission is infection of a child by the mother and diagonal transmission is the unproven concept of transmission of a virus from a father to a child, via the germ cells in, for instance, intracytoplasmic sperm injection (ICSI).

In this chapter, the current knowledge on the impact of HIV, HBV and HCV on male and female fertility is summarised and the available evidence on the effects on fertility of different kinds of therapy used to treat these infections is reviewed.

HIV and Semen Parameters

The HIV is spread via sexual contact, via the blood (products) and via vertical transmission. During an infection with HIV the number of CD4-positive lymphocytes, essential for cellular immunity, decreases and immunity against viruses and bacteria is reduced. Diseases that do not spread among people with normal immunity,

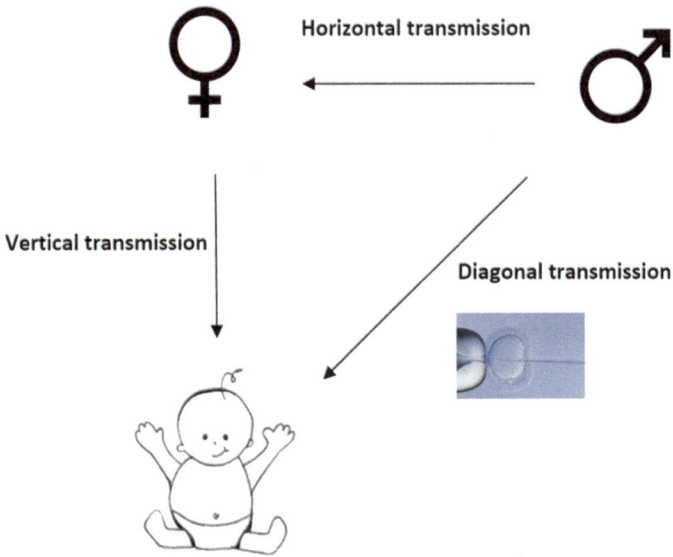

Fig. 1.1 Transmission after assisted reproductive techniques (ART)

the so-called opportunistic infections, can occur. This is known as acquired immunodeficiency syndrome (AIDS).

Unfortunately, at present, there is neither a cure nor a vaccination for HIV, and none is expected in the near future. The treatment of HIV consists of three antiviral agents, the so-called combination antiretroviral therapy (cART). The goal of cART is to suppress the virus and lower the amount of HIV RNA to undetectable levels. In the industrialised world, HIV became a chronic disease after the introduction of combination antiretroviral therapy (cART) in the mid-1990s. Therefore, it is now widely accepted that men and women infected with HIV, just like people with other chronic diseases, can become parents.

Sexual transmission remains the major route of transmission in couples who are serodiscordant for HIV, which means that one partner is infected with the disease and the other is not. In particular, HIV-negative women with an HIV-infected male partner are at risk of contracting HIV when they want to become pregnant because they have to avoid the use of a condom. The chance of HIV transmission is related to the amount of circulating HIV RNA [2]. In pregnant women the chance of vertical transmission of HIV is 0.5 % when HIV RNA levels are below detection limits at birth [3].

HIV in the Genital Tract

The HIV is present in the semen of asymptomatic men as cell-free HIV-RNA particles in seminal plasma and as a cell-associated virus in non-spermatozoal cells, such as lymphocytes and macrophages [4]. Most HIV-1 RNA seems to originate from the seminal vesicles and prostate, given that a vasectomy does not influence the concentration of HIV-1 RNA in semen [5]. Studies in the earlier days of HIV claim that HIV-1 DNA might be present in spermatozoa and spermatogonial stem cells [6–8], but later studies have contradicted these findings [9–11]. In addition, all studies but one report that the HIV-1 (co-) receptors CD4, CXCR4 and CCR5, which are necessary for the cellular entry of HIV-1, have not been demonstrated on the spermatozoal surface [12, 13]. Therefore, it seems unlikely that spermatozoa are directly infected with HIV-1 [9–11]. The finding that neither the partner nor the offspring was infected after semen-washing procedures, which are designed to separate spermatozoa from seminal plasma and to use the isolated spermatozoa for further fertility treatment, supports this theory [14].

During the first 20 years of the HIV/AIDS epidemic most gynaecologists were reluctant to accept HIV-serodiscordant couples in their infertility programmes [15–17]. Nowadays, serodiscordant couples with an HIV-infected man can adopt several strategies with the aim of impregnating the woman, which include:

1. Semen washing in combination with ART
2. Spontaneous conception while the man is successfully using cART
3. Spontaneous conception while the man is successfully using cART and the uninfected partner receives pre-exposure prophylaxis (PREP), which is called PREP for conception (PREP-C)

and can be given incidentally or daily. Most data are published on scenarios 1 and 2. There is no evidence at present that scenario 3, PREP-C, is more efficacious than cART alone.

Semen-washing protocols are aimed at separating the uninfected spermatozoa from the infectious seminal plasma. Semen-washing protocols differ between hospitals, but all procedures have a low sperm yield in common. When spermatozoa are frozen after processing and before insemination the sperm yield may be even lower. Furthermore, in most protocols some of the semen is used for polymerase chain reaction (PCR) testing after processing and even fewer spermatozoa can be used for insemination [18]. This implies artificial sterility for HIV-infected men, and only men with semen of good quality qualify for semen-washing and insemination. When there are not enough spermatozoa after washing, ICSI can be performed.

When using ICSI, there is a theoretical risk of the diagonal transmission of HIV. Indeed, integration of HIV into the genome was demonstrated in an in vitro study involving embryos from cats and rest embryos after in vitro fertilisation (IVF), but only at very high levels of HIV RNA [19]. In vivo, ICSI has been carried out without the partner or offspring becoming infected [14, 20]. Therefore, the theoretical chance of infecting a child via the paternal line, the so-called diagonal transmission, seems negligible, and ICSI is considered to be safe, especially at low levels of HIV RNA. It is thus important to know whether or not HIV affects semen quality.

In untreated HIV infection, the concentration of HIV RNA in semen is on average tenfold lower than that in blood plasma. Nevertheless, in some individuals the concentration of HIV-1-RNA in seminal plasma is higher than that in blood plasma. There are three explanations for this phenomenon:

1. The detection of distinct HIV-1 populations in the epididymis and prostate, other than in blood, suggests that HIV-1 particles can be produced locally in the male genital tract [21–23].
2. The composition of the ejaculate varies among men and over time in the same individual.
3. Local inflammation may increase HIV-1 RNA levels in semen, independent of HIV-1 RNA concentrations in blood [24, 25].

From cross-sectional and case-control studies, it appears that, in general, semen parameters are not impaired by asymptomatic HIV-infection [26–30], although some case–control studies reported that some semen parameters, i.e. concentration, volume and progressive motility, are impaired compared with HIV-negative men [31, 32]. The use of a case–control design may be questioned, as semen quality is very variable among the whole population, and for a patient it is not a question of whether or not his semen is of worse quality than that of his neighbour, but whether the duration of the disease or therapy impairs his semen quality.

Table 1.2 displays semen parameters of HIV-positive men. The fact that men with and without antiretroviral therapy were analysed as one group in most of these studies limits these results. It is therefore unclear whether the observed changes are caused by the HIV-1 infection itself or by the antiretroviral therapy. A decrease in semen volume and sperm motility was observed in a single semen donor, from whom multiple semen samples were available before and after seroconversion for HIV-1 [33]. Obviously, such observations are not available for larger patient numbers. A longitudinal study describing semen parameters during natural HIV-1 infection, with a follow-up period of 2 years, evaluated the effect of on-going HIV-1 infection on semen parameters. None of the semen parameters changed significantly during a follow-up period of 96 weeks; however, progressive motility was low at all time points, and semen volume was within the lower normal range, according to the World Health Organisation's 1999 criteria [34]. Impaired semen parameters are described below 200 cells/mm^3 or in men with AIDS [35].

cART and Semen Parameters

Most antiretrovirals penetrate well into the male genital tract, except for some protease inhibitors [4, 36], and in general, HIV-1 RNA concentrations in blood and seminal plasma show a parallel decrease in response to cART [36, 37]. However, discrepancies between HIV-1 RNA in blood and seminal plasma are occasionally

Table 1.2 Semen parameters in human immunodeficiency virus (HIV)-infected men

HIV	Design	Controls	Number of HIV+ men	Volume (mL)	Sperm concentration (10^6 per mL)	Total sperm number (10^6/ejaculate)	Progressive motility (a + b) (%)	Vitality (%)	Normal morphology (%)
WHO 2010 criteria				1.5	15	39	32	58	4
Pilatz et al. [29]	Cross-sectional	NA	116	2.4	42.4	75.2	41	76	4
Lambert-Niclot et al. [30]	Cross-sectional	NA	144	3.5	116	385	34	78.6	31
Kehl et al. [31]	Case-control	93 HIV−men of women with tubal infertility	133 100 cART, 33 no therapy	2.2	77	NM	51	NM	50
Nicopoullos et al. [109]	Cross-sectional	NA	426 samples	2.3	51.3	128.2	41.6	NM	25.8
Lorusso et al. [110]	Case-control	130 HIV−men	34 HIV+	2.5	24.7	NM	48	80	32
			41 HIV+/HCV+	3	22.3		46.4	75	31

(continued)

Table 1.2 (continued)

HIV	Design	Controls	Number of HIV+ men	Volume (mL)	Sperm concentration (10^6 per mL)	Total sperm number (10^6/ ejaculate)	Progressive motility (a + b) (%)	Vitality (%)	Normal morphology (%)
Van Leeuwen et al. [47]	Cohort	NA	34	2.1	77.5	179.2	28→17%↓	NM	43
Van Leeuwen et al. [34]	Cohort	NA	55	2.3	96	193.6	25↓	NM	44
Bujan et al. [32]	Case–control	216 HIV–men	190	3.3	108.3	330.9	39.2	68.8	27
Garrido et al. [111]	Cross-sectional	NA	27 HIV+ 46 HIV+/HCV+	3.7	78.4	136.1	45.3	NM	NM
Dulioust et al. [112]	Case–control	79 unselected HIV+ men 79 HIV– controls	189 men seeking ART 177 cART, 12 no therapy	3.3	96.7	298.3	38.4	73	40.4

Study	Design	Subjects							
Robbins et al. [35]	Cross-sectional	9 CD4<200	2.0→1.8	80.4→61.3	NM	20.9→34.1	72.6→79	32.8→33.8	
		11 CD4>200	1.5→2.3	52.3→128.5		10.6→11.5↓	44.6→66.5	22.1→29.4	
		Start cART or duotherapy							
Umapathy et al. [21]	No analysis, inclusion is biased by selecting infertile men in Africa								
Muller et al. [28]	Case–control	HIV–men	250	1.8	62	NM	52	NM	>35%
Dondero et al. [113]	Case–control	38 high-risk HIV–men	21	2.8	43	NM	22.5↓	NM	52
		30 HIV–men							
Politch et al. [114]	Cross-sectional	NA	166						
Crittenden et al. [26]	Case–control	51 HIV–men	39			48.8			
Krieger et al. [27]	Cross-sectional	NA	21 asymptomatic	2.5	109	285	62	NM	NM
		3 AIDS (50 samples)							

NA not applicable, NM not mentioned, cART combination antiretroviral therapy, HCV hepatitis C virus described. HIV-1 RNA can be detected in seminal plasma, despite adequate suppression of HIV-1 RNA in blood, and HIV-RNA can be detected from time to time in semen, despite stable levels or even undetectable levels of HIV-1 RNA in blood [12, 38–43].

In some countries, it is currently advocated that all people with HIV should start cART, irrespective of the immune status. The goal of this early treatment is twofold:

1. To minimise the risk of transmission to other people, as HIV-RNA concentrations decrease after cART is initiated, the so-called "treatment as prevention" [44]
2. To prevent HIV-related morbidity [45, 46]

As robust evidence is lacking that treatment for HIV above 500 CD4 cells/mm^3 is superior to treatment between 350 and 500 CD4 cells/mm^3 in relation to life expectancy and morbidities, this policy is not embraced in all countries and in those countries a more differentiated treatment is advocated; above 500 CD4 cells/mm^3 cART can be considered and at between 350 and 500 cells/mm^3, treatment should be initiated. In addition, it is estimated that people who are not aware of their HIV status transmit almost 90% of new infections during acute HIV infection.

It is as yet unknown whether or not this new policy of early treatment for HIV and the consequences of the long-term use of antiretrovirals will affect semen quality, but most studies conclude that semen parameters are stable under antiretroviral therapy [29].

Data on semen parameters before and after antiretroviral therapy are limited to those of three studies: semen parameters were normal according to WHO criteria and remained stable after the administration of zidovudine (AZT) monotherapy in five HIV-1 infected men [26], but improved in 20 men after 4 or 12 weeks of cART [35]. The observed improvement in the latter study may be caused by improved general health resulting from cART, as most patients had a low immunity. The follow-up in this study was too short to evaluate any potential detrimental impact of cART on spermatogenesis, because a full round of spermatogenesis takes ~70 days. Semen motility decreased after 48 weeks of cART from 28 to 17% [47]. One of the hypotheses put forward to explain the

possible decreased motility is that mitochondria might be negatively affected by cART [48].

Mitochondria are abundant in spermatozoa and necessary for
progressive motility. Deletions in mitochondrial DNA (mtDNA) of
spermatozoa have been described as a result of antiretroviral therapy [49]. Unfortunately, semen quality parameters were not analysed in this study. Theoretically, the penetration of nucleoside
reverse transcriptase inhibitors (NRTIs) into spermatozoa or their
precursors could result in mitochondrial toxicity and may lead to
impaired progressive motility. However, this hypothesis remains to
be proved and a more recent publication showed that spermatozoa
are not very suitable for testing mtDNA content [50].

It is not known at present if some cART regimes are more
harmful to spermatozoa than others. In general NRTIs penetrate
well into semen and protease inhibitors do not [51]. Nucleoside
analogues with proven mitochondrial toxicity in other tissues,
such as stavudine and didanosine, are no longer widely used and
less toxic regimes are prescribed. All studies on semen quality are
too small to distinguish between different kinds of cART. One
study speculated that nevirapine, which is only used for the treatment of people with low immunity, had fewer detrimental effects
than efavirenz [30].

Conception in HIV-Infected Men

Spontaneous conception in couples who are serodiscordant for
HIV is becoming increasingly acceptable. Vernazza et al. [52] published a protocol for PREP-C for HIV-discordant couples with a
positive male partner. PREP-C was later defined as "the use of
antiretroviral agents in the uninfected partner having timed unprotected sex with their HIV-1-positive man in an attempt to conceive
without HIV transmission" [53]. To reduce the risk of infection,
Vernazza proposed that the man or couple:

1. Should have been successfully treated with cART for more than
   6 months

2. Should have a stable relationship, and have no current symptoms of sexual transmitted diseases
3. Use a luteinising hormone (LH) test to determine the optimal timing of intercourse, i.e. 36 h after LH peak
4. Use tenofovir as PREP; the first dose at LH peak and the second dose 24 h later
5. Undergo a fertility evaluation after six attempts [52]

After a maximum of 12 attempts, 75 % of the 53 couples were pregnant. Recently, another PREP-C protocol was published. In this study, 8 on-going pregnancies were reported in 13 patients (62 %); this rate could become higher as couples who had only had one cycle of PREP-C were included and analysed [53]. As in the non-HIV-infected population, about 80 % of women conceive after 1 year, this could reflect normal fertility within a HIV-serodiscordant couple with a HIV-infected male partner [54].

The use of PREP-C is increasingly accepted and even advocated by the Centers for Disease Control (CDC) [55], but not all couples qualify for PREP-C, including women with hepatitis B/C; men with detectable HIV RNA in plasma and/or semen; sub-fertility and high anxiety regarding HIV transmission [53]. However, data are lacking if the additional use of PREP-C, in men in whom HIV RNA is undetectable using cART, is more effective than cART alone. Studies in which PREP-C is given on a daily basis, for at least 6 days before intercourse, show a larger efficacy than incidental PREP-C some hours before intercourse. Both daily tenofovir (TDF) and tenofovir–emtricitabine (FTC/TDF; Truvada®) are good agents for PREP [56].

Most heterosexual transmission studies do not qualify to study fertility, as pregnancy is not the primary endpoint, and in fact many women use contraceptives and couples use condoms. The drawback of PREP without known efficacy in men who are already being treated with cART is that the future fetus is being exposed to TDF alone or in combination with FTC (Truvada®), where the possible effects on the fetus are unknown. TDF and FTC/TDF, when used as PREP by HIV-1-uninfected men, did not adversely affect male fertility or pregnancy outcomes [57].

HIV and Female Fertility

Case–control studies have suggested lower pregnancy rates in HIV-1-infected women compared with women without HIV-1 infection, irrespective of past or current additional sexually transmitted disease (STD) [58, 59]. It was recently confirmed that even in the Western world, where cART is widely available and mother-to-child transmission (MTCT) rates are low, pregnancy rates were 40 % lower and time to pregnancy was 75 % longer amongst HIV-infected women compared with uninfected women [60]. It is unclear at present if these decreased pregnancy rates are caused by biological changes or by an alteration in sexual behaviour after HIV diagnosis [60]. On the other hand, pregnancy has no influence on the course of HIV [61].

There are some biological phenomena that may explain the lower pregnancy rates in HIV-infected women. First, cohort studies have demonstrated a high prevalence of STDs in HIV-1-infected women. These women may therefore also be at risk of tubal infertility [62, 63]. Second, menstrual cycle disturbances; polymenorrhoea and oligomenorrhoea, i.e. very short menstrual cycles or long menstrual cycles, which are associated with subfertility, are equally prevalent in asymptomatic HIV-1-infected women and in HIV-1-negative controls [64, 65], although more advanced immunodeficiency is associated with menstrual dysfunction [65]. Third, ovarian reserve may be impaired in HIV-infected women. HIV was considered an independent factor for early menopause and some claim a higher incidence of severe ovarian dysfunction [66]. Occasionally, a low anti-Müllerian hormone, (AMH) level, a high follicle-stimulating hormone (FSH) level or a low antral follicle count (AFC) as a marker of imminent ovarian failure was described [67–70]. However, markers for ovarian reserve are not very reliable for predicting spontaneous conception and their random use should be avoided [71].

In addition, outcomes of IVF in HIV-infected women are conflicting. Some show a similar response to IVF to HIV-negative women [69], whereas others claim that HIV-infected women under cART undergoing IVF have a lower pregnancy rate than non-infected controls [72]. It was hypothesised that mitochondrial toxicity caused by antiretrovirals might be the underlying mechanism of the low pregnancy rate, as oocytes from infertile, HIV-infected highly active antiretroviral therapy (HAART)-treated women show decreased mtDNA content [73], but this has not been confirmed in larger studies. Another ICSI study had similar pregnancy rates amongst HIV-infected women to matched HIV-negative controls, but stimulation was often cancelled because of a low response [74].

Progression of HIV-1 disease results in a dramatic decline in pregnancy and live birth rates [75]. cART reverses these changes and is associated with increased pregnancy rates in HIV-positive women, particularly those with higher CD4 counts and a good immunological response to therapy compared with untreated HIV-infected women [76, 77].

Conception in HIV-Infected Women

Women who are HIV-positive can practise self-insemination with no risk of infecting their HIV-negative partner. Recently, PREP-C has also been suggested for this population. It is encouraging, that the overall pregnancy incidence in HIV-1-infected female partners of HIV-negative men who used PREP was 12.9 per 100 person-years and did not differ significantly across the study arms (13.2 TDF, 12.4 FTC/TDF, 13.2 placebo). The frequencies of live births, pregnancy losses and gestational age at birth or loss were also statistically similar in the three randomisation groups [57].

Hepatitis B Characteristics

Hepatitis B is a liver infection that is caused by the hepatitis B virus (HBV), which is transmitted by vertical transmission, sexual contact and blood–blood contact. Chronic hepatitis B can lead to cirrhosis and hepatocellular carcinoma. All pregnant women and couples who undergo IVF or ICSI are tested for HBV and recipients of organs, including gametes or embryos, of HBV-positive carriers should all be vaccinated against HBV.

Hepatitis B seroconversion can occur spontaneously, but if not, the individual is said to have chronic disease , is therefore a carrier and can transmit HBV to their partner. The predominant way to transmit HBV is sexually and the rate of infection is dependent on the concentration of HBV DNA [78, 79]. With regard to highly infectious pregnant women, reflected by a positive hepatitis E antigen, vertical transmission occurs in up to 5% of cases, despite immunisation and vaccination of the neonate at birth [80]. In pregnancy, sometimes a short course of antivirals such as lamivudine or tenofovir, are given when viral loads are very high to prevent vertical transmission [81, 82].

In contrast to HIV, people who are infected with HBV or who test HBV-positive during a fertility workup only require ART when they have a fertility problem. Vice versa, pregnancy may delay hepatitis antigen seroconversion and may lead to more chronicity [83].

HBV and the Male Genital Tract

The HBV is present in semen as hepatitis B DNA (HBV DNA). The difference between HBV and HIV is that HBV not only passes through the blood–testis barrier, it is also thought to integrate into the genome of germ cells and cause damage [84]. In vitro studies show evidence of the integration of HBV DNA in oocytes and embryos via the maternal and paternal line [85]. Interestingly, the rate of integration was positively related to the level of HBV DNA [85]. Some claim that ICSI should be applied with caution in hepatitis B, because of the fear of the virus integrating into the developing embryo and thereby of HBV transmitting vertically or even diagonally via the germ cells, possibly resulting in a transfected embryo [86]. However, this has only been shown after IVF and in ICSI embryos and has never been studied in human embryos conceived naturally [85]. Although some report that HBV transmission is possible via the paternal germ cells, ultimate proof of this concept is lacking [87]. In fact, the difference between ICSI and IVF is in fact artificial, as the integration of HBV into the genome of the embryo also occurs in IVF; therefore, integration of HBV could in theory also occur in spontaneous conception. From mice studies it is clear that integration of HBV into the genome of the mice embryo does indeed take place, but no adverse effects are seen after ten generations of mice [88]. Some hospitals have an upper bound limit of viral load in which they accept patients for ICSI because of a fear of transfected embryos. Patients with higher HBV loads are then referred to their treating liver specialist for (temporary) treatment before ICSI is applied.

HBV and Male Fertility

Unfortunately, there are no studies that compare fertility or spontaneous conception rates in HBV-infected populations with noninfected populations. Studies on male fertility and HBV are limited to evaluating semen quality in HBV-infected men. It is of great importance to keep in mind that the quality of these studies is low, as they do not consist of an unselected population, but rather of men who had already required ART because of fertility problems in the couple.

Semen studies are shown in Table 1.3. In general, progressive motility was low compared with non-HBV-infected men. It is speculated that this could be caused by oxidative stress due to viral infections or chromosomal instability [86]. However, controls were not always matched, and in one study, for instance, the HBV group consisted of more men with male or unexplained infertility [89].

Conflicting results were reported in the outcomes of IVF treatments in couples with at least one HBV-seropositive partner. In one study, lower implantation and pregnancy rates were observed in HBV-positive individuals compared with healthy controls [90]. Another study, in contrast, reported higher implantation and pregnancy rates in the HBV-seropositive group [91]. Zhou et al. [92] suggested that HBV infection in men might be associated with poor sperm quality and worse ICSI and embryo transfer outcomes, but HBV did not affect the outcomes of IVF and embryo transfer.

Table 1.3 Semen parameters in hepatitis B (HBV)-infected men

HBV	Design	Controls	Number of HBV men	Volume (mL)	Sperm concentration (10^6 per mL)	Total sperm number (10^6/ejaculate)	Progressive motility (a+b) (%)	Vitality (%)	Normal morphology (%)
WHO 2010 criteria				1.5	15	39	32	58	4
Oger et al. [89]	Case control	HBV negative	32	NM	90	NM	36	66	38
Moretti et al. [115]	Case control	HBV, healthy control	13	NM	127	NM	31	NM	27
Lorusso et al. [110]	Case control	HCV. HIV healthy control	30	2.2	6.9↓	NM	37	73	27

Poor semen quality and a lower number of embryos were confirmed in another study, but no difference in clinical and on-going pregnancies was observed [89].

HBV and Female Fertility

To our knowledge, there are no studies that describe the fertility rates in unselected HBV-positive women. It was suggested that HBV-positive women might have inferior outcomes compared with non-infected women, but all women needed ART to overcome infertility [93]. Moreover, clinical pregnancy rates, a more important outcome, were similar in HBV and HBV groups [93]. Maternal hepatitis antigen carrier status did not add a risk of adverse neonatal outcomes or a detrimental effect on the child's growth; therefore, heightening surveillance for adverse neonatal complications in HBV-infected pregnant women may be unnecessary [94].

HCV Transmission

Hepatitis C virus (HCV) infection is an infection of the liver that could lead to cirrhosis and hepatocellular carcinoma. Traditionally, hepatitis C is a disease that is transmitted by blood products or intravenous drug use. The risk of sexual transmission is estimated to be 0.07% per year (95% CI: 0.01, 0.13) or 1 per 190,000 occurrences of intercourse in heterosexual couples [95]. There is no vaccination for HCV. Recently, trials were published in which HCV was successfully treated with new antiviral agents, although these treatments are not yet widely available [96]. The chance of vertical transmission in an HCV-positive pregnant woman is 2–6% [97].

Few data exist on fertility in random HCV-infected populations. Because the main route of hepatitis C transmission is not sexual contact, there is some debate whether or not HCV-infected men should use semen-washing procedures in combination with ART. In theory, the diagonal transmission of HCV is possible via ICSI. In HCV-positive men semen-washing procedures are performed with

ICSI to diminish the chance of horizontal and diagonal transmission. After semen-washing, HCV was no longer detectable, whereas HCV was detected in 20.4% of 153 samples before semen-washing [98]. With a risk of sexual transmission that is known to be very low, semen-washing procedures without testing after washing seem justified [99]. ICSI with semen-washing is performed for a prolonged period without any known cases of infection in the partner [99, 100]. ICSI in HIV-positive women did not lead to a higher infection rate in the offspring [101]. With the perspective of a cure for HCV, ART will no longer be necessary in overcoming HCV for this specific patient group, but will remain necessary for couples with HCV and infertility.

HCV and Male Fertility

Analogous to hepatitis B, most studies report on semen quality in an attempt to study fertility, as is displayed in Table 1.4. Again, it is sometimes not clear if men were already infertile when they enrolled in the studies. In general, semen parameters in hepatitis C are normal according to WHO 2010 criteria; in some studies, progressive motility was decreased. In a study that selected HCV-positive men with no history of infertility, the duration of HCV infection correlated negatively with semen volume and semen motility [102]. In this study, a low serum testosterone level was described [102]. It is speculated that HCV might stimulate oxidative stress, which causes impaired spermatogenesis in general and impaired motility in particular. It is unknown whether or not antiviral therapy can undo these changes [102].

Therapy for HCV and Male Fertility

Until a few years ago, ribavirin and peginterferon constituted the most effective treatment available for HCV, with a sustained response in 40–50% of patients. Because of embryo toxicity and teratogenic effects described in animal studies, partners of men on

Table 1.4 Semen parameters in HCV-infected men

HCV	Design	Controls	Number of HCV men	Volume (mL)	Sperm concentration (10^6 per mL)	Total sperm number (10^6/ejaculate)	Progressive motility (a+b) (%)	Vitality (%)	Normal morphology (%)
WHO 2010 criteria				1.5	15	39	32	58	4
Garrido et al. [111]	Case–control	HIV+, healthy controls	55	3.4	92	NM	46.1	NM	NM
Durazzo et al. [116]	Longitudinal cohort	Healthy controls	10	NM	85.5	NM	45.7	NM	28.1
Moretti et al. [115]	Case–control	HBV, healthy control	13	NM	83	NM	24↓	NM	23
Lorusso et al. [110]	Case–control	HBV. HIV healthy control	27	3	9.3↓	NM	44	70	25
Safarinejad et al. [117]	Case–control	Healthy controls	82	NM	NM	21.5↓	26.2↓	NM	8.2
Hofny et al. [102]	Case–control	Healthy controls	55	2.3	40.1	NM	39.6	NM	59.7
La Vignera et al. [118]	Case–control	Healthy controls	60	2.7	39.9	108	20.2↓	NM	12

ribavirin were advised to take contraceptives during therapy and women were advised to take contraceptives until 6 months after therapy [103, 104]. One case report that described the effects of ribavirin and peginterferon on semen quality reported decreased motility during treatment and DNA packaging abnormalities until 8 months after treatment, which would justify longer contraceptive use in the partners of men infected with HIV being treated with ribavirin [105]. To our knowledge, there are no studies that describe the effects of the newer antivirals on semen quality.

HCV and Female Fertility

It is unknown whether or not asymptomatic HCV infection affects female fertility. In advanced disease complicated by cirrhosis, many women are infertile because of amenorrhoea and anovulation [106]. However, for women with cirrhosis who do become pregnant, the risk of maternal and fetal complications is estimated to be around 50 % of cases and maternal mortality has been reported in up to 10 % of cases [106].

In IVF, women with HCV had a worse ovarian response, but pregnancy rates were similar [107]. Pregnancy rates after ICSI were decreased in HCV-infected women compared with HCV-negative women, with a higher impact on PCR-positive cases [108] It was speculated that the negative outcome in ICSI might be a result of hormonal disturbance associated with viral liver cirrhosis, coinciding with active viral replication [108].

Conclusion

Semen parameters are stable in asymptomatic HIV-1-infected men not on antiretroviral therapy, but spontaneous pregnancy rates seem to be reduced in HIV-1-infected women compared with HIV-1-negative women. The long-term effects of antiretroviral therapy on male and female fertility are unknown.

Whether or not fertility is impaired in HBV- and HCV-positive men and women remains controversial and the underlying mechanism needs further exploration..

HIV-1-infected patients desiring offspring can opt for several modes of reproduction, including various forms of ART. ART with semen-processing is effective in generating pregnancies and has been performed in HIV-1-infected couples since the early 1990s without any reported seroconversion. More data should be generated on spontaneous conception under cART. As there is no proof that PREP-C in combination with a partner on cART is more effective than cART alone, this strategy should be evaluated. Data on ART in HIV-infected women are scarce. More data should be generated on ART in HIV-infected women and prognostic factors in relation to the ART outcome of both HIV-1-infected men and women need to be identified. The concept of the diagonal transmission of the virus via the paternal germline deserves further exploration, to prevent transgenic offspring.

References

1. Kalu E, et al. Fertility needs and funding in couples with blood-borne viral infection. HIV Med. 2010;11(1):90–3.
2. Quinn TC, et al. Viral load and heterosexual transmission of human immunodeficiency virus type 1. Rakai Project Study Group. N Engl J Med. 2000;342(13):921–9.
3. Warszawski J, et al. Mother-to-child HIV transmission despite antiretroviral therapy in the ANRS French Perinatal Cohort. AIDS. 2008;22(2):289–99.
4. Lowe SH, et al. Is the male genital tract really a sanctuary site for HIV? Arguments that it is not. AIDS. 2004;18(10):1353–62.
5. Anderson DJ, et al. White blood cells and HIV-1 in semen from vasectomised seropositive men. Lancet. 1991;338(8766):573–4.
6. Nuovo GJ, et al. HIV-1 nucleic acids localize to the spermatogonia and their progeny. A study by polymerase chain reaction in situ hybridization. Am J Pathol. 1994;144(6):1142–8.
7. Bagasra O, et al. Detection of HIV-1 proviral DNA in sperm from HIV-1-infected men. AIDS. 1994;8(12):1669–74.

8. Scofield VL, et al. HIV interaction with sperm. AIDS. 1994;8(12):1733–6.

9. Quayle AJ, et al. The case against an association between HIV-1 and sperm: molecular evidence. J Reprod Immunol. 1998;41(1–2):127–36.

10. Quayle AJ, et al. T lymphocytes and macrophages, but not motile spermatozoa, are a significant source of human immunodeficiency virus in semen. J Infect Dis. 1997;176(4):960–8.

11. Pudney J, et al. Microscopic evidence against HIV-1 infection of germ cells or attachment to sperm. J Reprod Immunol. 1999;44(1–2): 57–77.

12. Kim LU, et al. Evaluation of sperm washing as a potential method of reducing HIV transmission in HIV-discordant couples wishing to have children. AIDS. 1999;13(6):645–51.

13. Muciaccia B, et al. HIV-1 chemokine co-receptor CCR5 is expressed on the surface of human spermatozoa. AIDS. 2005;19(13):1424–6.

14. Vitorino RL, et al. Systematic review of the effectiveness and safety of assisted reproduction techniques in couples serodiscordant for human immunodeficiency virus where the man is positive. Fertil Steril. 2011;95(5):1684–90.

15. Sauer MV. Providing fertility care to those with HIV: time to re-examine healthcare policy. Am J Bioeth. 2003;3(1):33–40.

16. Anderson DJ, Politch JA. Providing fertility care to HIV-1 serodiscordant couples: a biologist's point of view. Am J Bioeth. 2003;3(1):47–9.

17. Bendikson KA, Anderson D, Hornstein MD. Fertility options for HIV patients. Curr Opin Obstet Gynecol. 2002;14(5):453–7.

18. Pasquier C, et al. Multicenter assessment of HIV-1 RNA quantitation in semen in the CREAThE network. J Med Virol. 2012;84(2):183–7.

19. Steenvoorden MM, et al. Integration of immunodeficiency virus in oocytes via intracytoplasmic injection: possible but extremely unlikely. Fertil Steril. 2012;98(1):173–7.

20. Sauer MV, et al. Providing fertility care to men seropositive for human immunodeficiency virus: reviewing 10 years of experience and 420 consecutive cycles of in vitro fertilization and intracytoplasmic sperm injection. Fertil Steril. 2009;91(6):2455–60.

21. Umapathy E, et al. Sperm characteristics and accessory sex gland functions in HIV-infected men. Arch Androl. 2001;46(2):153–8.

22. Paranjpe S, et al. Subcompartmentalization of HIV-1 quasispecies between seminal cells and seminal plasma indicates their origin in distinct genital tissues. AIDS Res Hum Retroviruses. 2002;18(17):1271–80.

23. Coombs RW, Reichelderfer PS, Landay AL. Recent observations on HIV type-1 infection in the genital tract of men and women. AIDS. 2003;17(4):455–80.

24. Cohen MS, et al. Reduction of concentration of HIV-1 in semen after treatment of urethritis: implications for prevention of sexual transmission of HIV-1. AIDSCAP Malawi Research Group. Lancet. 1997;349(9069):1868–73.

25. Ping LH, et al. Effects of genital tract inflammation on human immunodeficiency virus type 1 V3 populations in blood and semen. J Virol. 2000;74(19):8946–52.

26. Crittenden JA, Handelsman DJ, Stewart GJ. Semen analysis in human immunodeficiency virus infection. Fertil Steril. 1992;57(6):1294–9.

27. Krieger JN, et al. Fertility parameters in men infected with human immunodeficiency virus. J Infect Dis. 1991;164(3):464–9.

28. Muller CH, Coombs RW, Krieger JN. Effects of clinical stage and immunological status on semen analysis results in human immunodeficiency virus type 1-seropositive men. Andrologia. 1998;30 Suppl 1:15–22.

29. Pilatz A, et al. Semen quality in HIV patients under stable antiretroviral therapy is impaired compared to WHO 2010 reference values and on sperm proteome level. AIDS. 2014;28(6):875–80.

30. Lambert-Niclot S, et al. Effect of antiretroviral drugs on the quality of semen. J Med Virol. 2011;83(8):1391–4.

31. Kehl S, et al. HIV-infection and modern antiretroviral therapy impair sperm quality. Arch Gynecol Obstet. 2011;284(1):229–33.

32. Bujan L, et al. Decreased semen volume and spermatozoa motility in HIV-1-infected patients under antiretroviral treatment. J Androl. 2007;28(3):444–52.

33. van Leeuwen E, et al. Semen parameters of a semen donor before and after infection with human immunodeficiency virus type 1: case report. Hum Reprod. 2004;19(12):2845–8.

34. van Leeuwen E, et al. Semen quality remains stable during 96 weeks of untreated human immunodeficiency virus-1 infection. Fertil Steril. 2008;90(3):636–41.

35. Robbins WA, et al. Antiretroviral therapy effects on genetic and morphologic end points in lymphocytes and sperm of men with human immunodeficiency virus infection. J Infect Dis. 2001;184(2):127–35.

36. Taylor S, Pereira AS. Antiretroviral drug concentrations in semen of HIV-1 infected men. Sex Transm Infect. 2001;77(1):4–11.

37. Barroso PF, et al. Effect of antiretroviral therapy on HIV shedding in semen. Ann Intern Med. 2000;133(4):280–4.

38. Zhang H, et al. Human immunodeficiency virus type 1 in the semen of men receiving highly active antiretroviral therapy. N Engl J Med. 1998;339(25):1803–9.
39. Gupta P, et al. Human immunodeficiency virus type 1 shedding pattern in semen correlates with the compartmentalization of viral Quasi species between blood and semen. J Infect Dis. 2000;182(1):79–87.
40. Vernazza PL, et al. Potent antiretroviral treatment of HIV-infection results in suppression of the seminal shedding of HIV. The Swiss HIV Cohort Study. AIDS. 2000;14(2):117–21.
41. Bujan L, et al. Intermittent human immunodeficiency type 1 virus (HIV-1) shedding in semen and efficiency of sperm processing despite high seminal HIV-1 RNA levels. Fertil Steril. 2002;78(6):1321–3.
42. Leruez-Ville M, et al. Assisted reproduction in HIV-1-serodifferent couples: the need for viral validation of processed semen. AIDS. 2002;16(17):2267–73.
43. Bujan L, et al. Factors of intermittent HIV-1 excretion in semen and efficiency of sperm processing in obtaining spermatozoa without HIV-1 genomes. AIDS. 2004;18(5):757–66.
44. Cohen MS, et al. Prevention of HIV-1 infection with early antiretroviral therapy. N Engl J Med. 2011;365(6):493–505.
45. Grinsztejn B, et al. Effects of early versus delayed initiation of antiretroviral treatment on clinical outcomes of HIV-1 infection: results from the phase 3 HPTN 052 randomised controlled trial. Lancet Infect Dis. 2014;14(4):281–90.
46. Kitahata MM, et al. Effect of early versus deferred antiretroviral therapy for HIV on survival. N Engl J Med. 2009;360(18): 1815–26.
47. van Leeuwen E, et al. Effects of antiretroviral therapy on semen quality. AIDS. 2008;22(5):637–42.
48. Vernazza P. HAART improves quality of life: should we care about the quality of spermatozoa? AIDS. 2008;22(5):647–8.
49. White AJ. Mitochondrial toxicity and HIV therapy. Sex Transm Infect. 2001;77(3):158–73.
50. Diehl S, et al. Mitochondrial DNA and sperm quality in patients under antiretroviral therapy. AIDS. 2003;17(3):450–1.
51. Else LJ, et al. Pharmacokinetics of antiretroviral drugs in anatomical sanctuary sites: the male and female genital tract. Antivir Ther. 2011;16(8):1149–67.
52. Vernazza PL, et al. Preexposure prophylaxis and timed intercourse for HIV-discordant couples willing to conceive a child. AIDS. 2011;25(16):2005–8.

53. Whetham J, et al. Pre-exposure prophylaxis for conception (PrEP-C) as a risk reduction strategy in HIV-positive men and HIV-negative women in the UK. AIDS Care. 2014;26(3):332–6.

54. Gnoth C, et al. Time to pregnancy: results of the German prospective study and impact on the management of infertility. Hum Reprod. 2003;18(9):1959–66.

55. Centers for Disease Control and Prevention. Interim guidance for clinicians considering the use of preexposure prophylaxis for the prevention of HIV infection in heterosexually active adults. MMWR Morb Mortal Wkly Rep. 2012;61(31):586–9.

56. Baeten JM, et al. Antiretroviral prophylaxis for HIV prevention in heterosexual men and women. N Engl J Med. 2012;367(5): 399–410.

57. Were EO, et al. Pre-exposure prophylaxis does not affect the fertility of HIV-1-uninfected men. AIDS. 2014;28(13):1977–82.

58. Gregson S, Zaba B, Garnett GP. Low fertility in women with HIV and the impact of the epidemic on orphanhood and early childhood mortality in sub-Saharan Africa. AIDS. 1999;13(Suppl A):S249–57.

59. Lo JC, Schambelan M. Reproductive function in human immunodeficiency virus infection. J Clin Endocrinol Metab. 2001;86(6): 2338–43.

60. Linas BS, et al. Relative time to pregnancy among HIV-infected and uninfected women in the Women's Interagency HIV Study, 2002-2009. AIDS. 2011;25(5):707–11.

61. Saada M, et al. Pregnancy and progression to AIDS: results of the French prospective cohorts. SEROGEST and SEROCO Study Groups. AIDS. 2000;14(15):2355–60.

62. Frankel RE, et al. High prevalence of gynecologic disease among hospitalized women with human immunodeficiency virus infection. Clin Infect Dis. 1997;25(3):706–12.

63. Sobel JD. Gynecologic infections in human immunodeficiency virus-infected women. Clin Infect Dis. 2000;31(5):1225–33.

64. Chirgwin KD, et al. Menstrual function in human immunodeficiency virus-infected women without acquired immunodeficiency syndrome. J Acquir Immune Defic Syndr Hum Retrovirol. 1996;12(5):489–94.

65. Harlow SD, et al. Effect of HIV infection on menstrual cycle length. J Acquir Immune Defic Syndr. 2000;24(1):68–75.

66. Schoenbaum EE, et al. HIV infection, drug use, and onset of natural menopause. Clin Infect Dis. 2005;41(10):1517–24.

67. Clark RA, et al. Frequency of anovulation and early menopause among women enrolled in selected adult AIDS clinical trials group studies. J Infect Dis. 2001;184(10):1325–7.

68. Englert Y, et al. Medically assisted reproduction in the presence of chronic viral diseases. Hum Reprod Update. 2004;10(2):149–62.
69. Martinet V, et al. Ovarian response to stimulation of HIV-positive patients during IVF treatment: a matched, controlled study. Hum Reprod. 2006;21(5):1212–7.
70. Ohl J, et al. [Alterations of ovarian reserve tests in Human Immunodeficiency Virus (HIV)-infected women]. Gynecol Obstet Fertil. 2010;38(5):313–7.
71. Tremellen K, Savulescu J. Ovarian reserve screening: a scientific and ethical analysis. Hum Reprod. 2014;29(12):2606–14.
72. Ohl J, et al. Assisted reproduction techniques for HIV serodiscordant couples: 18 months of experience. Hum Reprod. 2003;18(6):1244–9.
73. Lopez S, et al. Mitochondrial DNA depletion in oocytes of HIV-infected antiretroviral-treated infertile women. Antivir Ther. 2008;13(6):833–8.
74. Terriou P, et al. Outcome of ICSI in HIV-1-infected women. Hum Reprod. 2005;20(10):2838–43.
75. Sedgh G, et al. HIV-1 disease progression and fertility in Dar es Salaam, Tanzania. J Acquir Immune Defic Syndr. 2005;39(4):439–45.
76. Myer L, et al. Impact of antiretroviral therapy on incidence of pregnancy among HIV-infected women in Sub-Saharan Africa: a cohort study. PLoS Med. 2010;7(2):e1000229.
77. Makumbi FE, et al. Associations between HIV antiretroviral therapy and the prevalence and incidence of pregnancy in Rakai, Uganda. AIDS Res Treat. 2011;2011:519492.
78. Centers for Disease Control and Prevention. Updated CDC recommendations for the management of hepatitis B virus-infected healthcare providers and students. MMWR Recomm Rep. 2012;61(RR-3):1–12.
79. Incident Investigation Teams and Others, et al. Transmission of hepatitis B to patients from four infected surgeons without hepatitis B e antigen. N Engl J Med. 1997;336(3):178–84.
80. Lin X, et al. Immunoprophylaxis failure against vertical transmission of hepatitis B virus in the Chinese population: a hospital-based study and a meta-analysis. Pediatr Infect Dis J. 2014;33(9):897–903.
81. Jackson V, et al. Lamivudine treatment and outcome in pregnant women with high hepatitis B viral loads. Eur J Clin Microbiol Infect Dis. 2015;34(3):619–23.
82. Greenup AJ, et al. Efficacy and safety of tenofovir disoproxil fumarate in pregnancy to prevent perinatal transmission of hepatitis B virus. J Hepatol. 2014;61(3):502–7.
83. Han YT, et al. Clinical features and outcome of acute hepatitis B in pregnancy. BMC Infect Dis. 2014;14:368.

84. Huang JM, et al. Effects of hepatitis B virus infection on human sperm chromosomes. World J Gastroenterol. 2003;9(4):736–40.
85. Hu XL, et al. The presence and expression of the hepatitis B virus in human oocytes and embryos. Hum Reprod. 2011;26(7):1860–7.
86. Garolla A, et al. Sperm viral infection and male infertility: focus on HBV, HCV, HIV, HPV, HSV, HCMV, and AAV. J Reprod Immunol. 2013;100(1):20–9.
87. Ye F, et al. [Relationship between the expression of HBV mRNA in embryos and father-to-infant HBV transmission]. Zhonghua Nan Ke Xue. 2013;19(5):429–33.
88. Bagis H, et al. Stable transmission and expression of the hepatitis B virus total genome in hybrid transgenic mice until F10 generation. J Exp Zool A Comp Exp Biol. 2006;305(5):420–7.
89. Oger P, et al. Adverse effects of hepatitis B virus on sperm motility and fertilization ability during IVF. Reprod Biomed Online. 2011;23(2):207–12.
90. Pirwany IR, et al. Reproductive performance of couples discordant for hepatitis B and C following IVF treatment. J Assist Reprod Genet. 2004;21(5):157–61.
91. Lam PM, et al. Hepatitis B infection and outcomes of in vitro fertilization and embryo transfer treatment. Fertil Steril. 2010;93(2):480–5.
92. Zhou XP, et al. Comparison of semen quality and outcome of assisted reproductive techniques in Chinese men with and without hepatitis B. Asian J Androl. 2011;13(3):465–9.
93. Shi L, et al. Hepatitis B virus infection reduces fertilization ability during in vitro fertilization and embryo transfer. J Med Virol. 2014;86(7):1099–104.
94. Chen J, et al. Minimal adverse influence of maternal hepatitis B carrier status on perinatal outcomes and child's growth. J Matern Fetal Neonatal Med. 2015;28(18):2192–6.
95. Terrault NA, et al. Sexual transmission of hepatitis C virus among monogamous heterosexual couples: the HCV partners study. Hepatology. 2013;57(3):881–9.
96. Sulkowski MS, Jacobson IM, Nelson DR. Daclatasvir plus sofosbuvir for HCV infection. N Engl J Med. 2014;370(16):1560–1.
97. Hurtado CW, et al. Innate immune function in placenta and cord blood of hepatitis C—seropositive mother-infant dyads. PLoS One. 2010;5(8):e12232.
98. Bourlet T, et al. Prospective evaluation of the threat related to the use of seminal fractions from hepatitis C virus-infected men in assisted reproductive techniques. Hum Reprod. 2009;24(3):530–5.

99. Savasi V, et al. Should HCV discordant couples with a seropositive male partner be treated with assisted reproduction techniques (ART)? Eur J Obstet Gynecol Reprod Biol. 2013;167(2):181–4.

100. Mencaglia L, et al. ICSI for treatment of human immunodeficiency virus and hepatitis C virus-serodiscordant couples with infected male partner. Hum Reprod. 2005;20(8):2242–6.

101. Nesrine F, Saleh H. Hepatitis C virus (HCV) status in newborns born to HCV positive women performing intracytoplasmic sperm injection. Afr Health Sci. 2012;12(1):58–62.

102. Hofny ER, et al. Semen and hormonal parameters in men with chronic hepatitis C infection. Fertil Steril. 2011;95(8):2557–9.

103. Narayana K, D'Souza UJ, Rao KP. Effect of ribavirin on epididymal sperm count in rat. Indian J Physiol Pharmacol. 2002;46(1):97–101.

104. Narayana K, D'Souza UJ, Seetharama Rao KP. Ribavirin-induced sperm shape abnormalities in Wistar rat. Mutat Res. 2002; 513(1–2):193–6.

105. Pecou S, et al. Ribavirin and pegylated interferon treatment for hepatitis C was associated not only with semen alterations but also with sperm deoxyribonucleic acid fragmentation in humans. Fertil Steril. 2009;91(3):933.e17–22.

106. Ellington SR, et al. Recent trends in hepatic diseases during pregnancy in the United States, 2002-2010. Am J Obstet Gynecol. 2014;212(4):524.e1–7.

107. Englert Y, et al. Impaired ovarian stimulation during in vitro fertilization in women who are seropositive for hepatitis C virus and seronegative for human immunodeficiency virus. Fertil Steril. 2007;88(3):607–11.

108. Hanafi NF, Abo Ali AH, Abo el kheir HF. ICSI outcome in women who have positive PCR result for hepatitis C virus. Hum Reprod. 2011;26(1):143–7.

109. Nicopoullos JD, et al. A decade of the sperm-washing programme: correlation between markers of HIV and seminal parameters. HIV Med. 2011;12(4):195–201.

110. Lorusso F, et al. Impact of chronic viral diseases on semen parameters. Andrologia. 2010;42(2):121–6.

111. Garrido N, et al. Semen characteristics in human immunodeficiency virus (HIV)- and hepatitis C (HCV)-seropositive males: predictors of the success of viral removal after sperm washing. Hum Reprod. 2005;20(4):1028–34.

112. Dulioust E, et al. Semen alterations in HIV-1 infected men. Hum Reprod. 2002;17(8):2112–8.

113. Dondero F, et al. Semen analysis in HIV seropositive men and in subjects at high risk for HIV infection. Hum Reprod. 1996;11(4):765–8.

114. Politch JA, et al. The effects of disease progression and zidovudine therapy on semen quality in human immunodeficiency virus type 1 seropositive men. Fertil Steril. 1994;61(5):922–8.

115. Moretti E, et al. Sperm ultrastructure and meiotic segregation in a group of patients with chronic hepatitis B and C. Andrologia. 2008;40(3):173–8.

116. Durazzo M, et al. Alterations of seminal and hormonal parameters: an extrahepatic manifestation of HCV infection? World J Gastroenterol. 2006;12(19):3073–6.

117. Safarinejad MR, Kolahi AA, Iravani S. Evaluation of semen variables, sperm chromosomal abnormalities and reproductive endocrine profile in patients with chronic hepatitis C. BJU Int. 2010;105(1):79–86.

118. La Vignera S, et al. Sperm DNA damage in patients with chronic viral C hepatitis. Eur J Intern Med. 2012;23(1):e19–24.

Chapter 2
HBV Virus in the Future

Giangulielmo Zehender, Erika Ebranati, Lisa Fiaschi, Massimo Ciccozzi, and Massimo Galli

Introduction

Hepatitis B virus (HBV) is a major health problem and chronically infects an estimated 240 million people worldwide [1]. There are approximately 620,000 HBV-related deaths and 4.5 million new HBV infections each year throughout the world. In highly endemic areas such as the central Asian republics, south-eastern Asia, sub-Saharan Africa and the Amazon basin, the HBV carrier rate is >8 %, whereas the prevalence of hepatitis B surface antigen (HBsAg) is <2 % in less endemic regions such as the United States, northern Europe, Australia and parts of South America. The Middle East, some eastern European countries and the Mediterranean basin are considered areas of intermediate endemicity, with carrier rates of between 2 and 8 % [1].

G. Zehender, PhD (✉) • E. Ebranati, PhD • L. Fiaschi • M. Galli
Dipartimento di Scienze Cliniche e Biomediche "Luigi Sacco",
Sezione di Malattie Infettive, Università degli Studi di Milano, Milan, Italy
e-mail: gianguglielmo.zehender@unimi.it

M. Ciccozzi, MD, PhD
Dipartimento Malattie Infettive, Parassitarie ed Immunomediate,
Istituto Superiore di Sanità, Rome, Italy

© Springer International Publishing Switzerland 2016
A. Borini, V. Savasi (eds.), *Assisted Reproductive
Technologies and Infectious Diseases*,
DOI 10.1007/978-3-319-30112-9_2

Despite the recent decrease in the rate of new cases, about 7000–8000 new diagnoses are made every year in Europe. The prevalence of HBV infection in Europe varies widely, but is generally higher in south-eastern than in north-western countries. The highest prevalence rates are in Turkey, Romania, Bulgaria, Greece, Albania and southern Italy [2].

The HBV is an enveloped DNA virus with a diameter of 42 nm (the so-called "Dane particle"), which belongs to the *Hepadnaviridae* family, and infects the hepatocytes of a wide range of animals belonging to several classes of birds (genus *Avihepadnavirus*) and mammals (genus *Orthohepadnavirus*). In particular, avian hepadnaviruses have been isolated from various species of ducks, geese, herons, storks, cranes and parrots [3], and orthohepadnaviruses have been discovered in rodents (squirrels, woodchucks), non-human primates (chimpanzees, gorillas, orangutans, gibbons and woolly monkeys) and, more recently, in bats from Myanmar [4].

The double-layered lipoprotein membrane derived from the infected cells making up the viral envelope contains the surface antigen (HBsAg), a mixture of small (S), medium (PreS2 and S) and large (PreS1, PreS2 and S) proteins that can also be observed circulating freely in the blood of infected subjects as 22-nm spherical and tubular particles.

The role of the S protein in virus attachment has not been conclusively demonstrated; however, this protein contains the major site for the binding of neutralising antibody, designated the *a* determinant. Two other major determinants of the S protein have also been described; one has either "d" or "y" specificity and the other has "w" or "r". All combinations of these determinants have been found, resulting in four major subtypes: adw, adr, ayw and ayr and nine minor subtypes, determined by mutually exclusive amino acids substitution in the S region of HBV DNA. Antibodies to the *a* determinant confer protection to all of these serotypes, whereas antibodies to the subtype determinants do not [5].

The viral nucleocapsid consists of the core protein (HBcAg) and encloses a single molecule of the viral genome. It consists of a small and circular partially double-stranded DNA of about 3.2 kb whose minus strand, which encompasses four partially overlapping genes (PreS/S, PreC/C, P and X) encoding for at least seven proteins, is incomplete. In particular, the three surface glycoproteins (the small S protein, the middle PreS2 and S protein and the largest Pre S1/PreS2 and S protein), two core antigens (HBcAg and HBeAg), the polymerase and the X protein, a small regulatory protein that is essential for in vivo viral replication [6]. It also plays a central role in hepatocarcinogenesis [7].

After attaching to a hepatocyte as a result of the binding of Pre-S1 with a still unknown specific cell receptor, the viral nucleic acid is transferred to the cell nucleus, where it is completed by cell polymerases and forms covalently closed circular DNA (cccDNA) [8]. This mainly non-integrated cccDNA acts as a template for the production of the four viral transcripts that are necessary for protein production, including an over-length "pre-genomic RNA" (pg-RNA) that gives rise to the core proteins and the viral genome.

After encapsidation, a molecule of pg-RNA is transformed by the viral reverse transcriptase into partially double-stranded circular genomic DNA, and the pg-RNA is degraded by the RNase-H activity of the P protein. Some of the newly produced capsids are not transferred to the cell surface, but return to the nucleus and contribute to the cccDNA reserve [8]. The production of the three surface proteins ensures virion secretion.

In spite of the constrained nature of its genetic evolution, which is due to the partial overlapping of the viral genes [9], the HBV genome is characterised by considerable variability because of the use of an RNA intermediate and reverse transcriptase during replication.

HBV Mutants

Mutations in the HBV genome can occur because of spontaneous errors of viral polymerase, and the action of pressure by the host immune system or by exogenous factors, including passive and/or active immunisation and drug treatment. HBV has a higher frequency of mutations than other DNA viruses because the virus replicates via an RNA intermediate, using a reverse transcriptase that lacks a proof-reading function such as the reverse transcriptase and RNA polymerases of other highly variance viruses. Mutations have been identified in all four HBV genes, but have been most fully characterised in the preC/C gene, the polymerase gene and the preS/S gene [10–12].

Basal Core Promoter, Pre-C/C Gene Mutants

Two major groups of mutations that result in reduced or blocked HBeAg expression have been identified. The most common mutation in the ORF pre-C/C region is a guanine to adenine substitution at nt position 1896 (G1896A) that results in a translational stop codon (TGG to TAG; TAG=stop codon). This codon stops the expression of the *e* protein, which is processed to produce HBeAg [13]. However, HBV DNA synthesis persists and may cause liver damage, with progression to cirrhosis and cancer. Loss of HBeAg expression can also occur with mutations in the basal core promoter (BCP) region that regulates the expression of both HBeAg and core protein [14]. These mutations have been associated with fulminant hepatitis and severe chronic liver disease [15, 16]. However, fulminant hepatitis can occur in the absence of such mutations [17, 18]. Additional studies are needed to determine the pathogenic basis and clinical sequelae arising from the selection of these mutants [12].

X Gene Mutations

As the X ORF overlaps the BCP completely, promoter mutations can affect the amino acids sequence of the X protein. The most common BCP double mutations occurring at nt 1762 (A1762T) and at nt 1764 (G1764A) can cause changes in the X protein that may affect its ability to transactivate the BCP. In addition, insertions or deletions in the BCP often shift the X gene frame, resulting in truncated forms of the X protein. These shortened X proteins lack the domain in the C terminus that is required for the transactivation activity of HBx antigen [10–12].

Polymerase Gene Mutants

Mutations of the polymerase gene have been associated with resistance to treatment with nucleoside/nucleotides analogues and with viral persistence [10–12, 19, 20]. The most common of these mutations occur at codon 528 (the template binding site of the polymerase) and at codon 552 of the tyrosine, methionine, aspartate, aspartate (YMDD) motif (the catalytic site of the polymerase).

Polymerase mutations have been demonstrated to emerge in up 80 % of patients after treatment with nucleoside/nucleotide analogues. These mutations significantly decrease the efficacy of treatment [21]. As the genome of HBV is organised into overlapping reading frames, the selection of polymerase mutants, favouring resistance, can result in the emergence of changes in the overlapping S-gene during long-term antiviral therapy, potentially altering its immunoreactivity [22, 23].

PreS/S Gene Mutants

Isolates with pre-S deletions are often found. There is evidence that a set of mutations (deletion in the pre-S region and in pre-core and BCP mutations) are significantly associated with progressive liver disease and hepatocellular carcinoma (HCC) [24].

Mutations in the S gene can lead to conformational changes in the *a* determinant, which is located between amino acids 124 and 147 of HBsAg and has a double-loop structure projecting from the surface of the virus; the second loop (amino acids 139–147) is the major target for neutralising anti-HBs.

The prototype of such mutants, the so-called G145R, which shows a point mutation from guanosine to adenosine at nucleotide position 587, resulting in an amino acid substitution from glycine (G) to arginine (R) at position 145 in the *a* determinant of the surface antigen, was first observed in Italy some 25 years ago [25]. This mutant has been shown to be infectious in experimentally infected chimpanzees [26]. Besides the G145R, other S-gene mutants across the entire *a* determinant region have been found worldwide. Concern has been expressed that these mutated viruses may allow replication of HBV in the presence of vaccine-induced anti-HBs or anti-HBs contained in hepatitis B immune globulin (HBIG; immunisation escape mutants). In addition, these mutants may not be detected by some commercially available HBsAg assays based on antibodies to the wild-type virus (diagnostic escape mutants) [27, 28].

Hepatitis B infection with S mutant viruses has been reported to occur in the presence of protective levels of anti-HBs in infants born to HBV-infected mothers who received prophylaxis with HBIG and/or hepatitis B vaccine [25, 29–32] in children who responded to vaccination [33], and in liver transplant recipients who received HBIG for the prophylaxis of relapse of the HBV infection [34]. However, in population-based studies of infants born to HBsAg-positive mothers, S-gene mutant viruses have not been found to be associated with a failure to prevent perinatal HBV transmission [35]. In addition, pre-exposure vaccination of chimpanzees with currently licensed vaccines (not containing pre-S epitopes) conferred protection after intravenous challenge with the G145R HBV [36, 37]. At present, no evidence exists that S-gene mutants have spread in immunised populations or that these mutants pose a threat to hepatitis B immunisation programmes [38]. Further studies and enhanced surveillance to detect the emergence of these mutants and those caused by the onset of resistance to the viral therapy (see above) are a high priority in monitoring the effectiveness of current immunisation strategies.

Hepatitis B surface antigen escape mutants, which cannot be detected by currently available HBsAg assays, are possible carriers of occult HBV infection (OBI) [39].

HBV Genotypes

On the basis of the sequence divergence established by analysing the entire viral genome, HBV has been classified into nine genotypes (A–I) and various subgenotypes (indicated by numbers), with a mean nucleotide difference of $\geq 8\%$ between genotypes and $\geq 4\%$ between subgenotypes, partially corresponding to the previously described serologically defined subtypes [40].

Hepatitis B virus genotypes have a characteristic ethnogeographic distribution. Some are ubiquitous, such as genotype A, which is present in north-western Europe, North America and Central Africa [40], and genotype D, which has been found throughout the world, although its highest prevalence is in the Mediterranean area, the Middle East and southern Asia, particularly India. Genotypes B and C are only present in Asia; genotype E is found in sub-Saharan Africa [40] and genotype F in South and Central America [40]. Genotype G has been found in France and the USA [41], whereas genotype H seems to be confined to the northern part of Latin America (Table 2.1) [42].

Table 2.1 Subgenotypes, subtypes and geographical origin of HBV

	Subgenotype	Subtype	Geographical origin
A	A1 (Aa, A′)	adw2, ayw1	Africa, Asia, South America
	A2 (Ae, A-A′)	adw2, ayw1	Northern Europe, North America, South Africa
	A3 (Ac)		Cameroon, Gabon, Rwanda
	A4		Mali, Gambia
	A5		Nigeria, Rwanda, Cameroon, Haiti (African population)
	A6		Congo, Rwanda
	A7	ayw1, adw2, ay	Cameroon, Rwanda
B	B1 (Bj)	adw2	Japan
	B2 (Ba)	adw2, adw3	Asia without Japan
	B3	adw2, ayw1	Indonesia, Philippines
	B4	ayw1, adw2	Vietnam, Cambodia
	B5		Philippines
	B6		Alaska, Northern Canada, Greenland
	B7-B9		Indonesia
C	C1 (Cs)	adrq+, ayr, adw2, ayw1	South East Asia (Vietnam, Myanmar, Thailand, Southern China)
	C2 (Ce)	adrq+, ayr	Far East (Korea, Japan, Northern China)
	C3	adrq−, adrq+	Pacific Islands (Micronesia, Melanesia, Polynesia)
	C4		Australia
	C5		Philippines, Vietnam
	C6		Indonesia, Philippines
	C7		Philippines
	C8-C16		Indonesia

(continued)

Table 2.1 (continued)

	Subgenotype	Subtype	Geographical origin
D	D1	ayw2, adw1, ayw1	Europe, Middle East, Asia, Tunisia, Egypt
	D2	ayw3, ayw1	Europe, Morocco, India
	D3	ayw3, ayw2, ayw4	South Africa, Asia, Europe, USA, Northern Canada
	D4	ayw2, ayw3	Australia, Japan, Papua New Guinea
	D5		East India, Japan
	D6		Indonesia
	D7		Tunisia
	D8		Niger
	D9		Eastern India
E		ayw4, ayw2	Sub-Saharan Africa, UK, France, Saudi Arabia
F	F1a	adw4, ayw4	South and Central America
	F1b	adw4	Argentina, Japan, Venezuela, USA
	F2	adw4	South America (Brazil, Venezuela, Nicaragua)
	F3	adw4	Venezuela, Panama, Columbia, Bolivia
	F4	adw4	Bolivia, France, Argentina
G		adw2	USA, Germany, Japan, France, Mexico
H		adw4	USA, Japan, Nicaragua
I	I1	adw2	Laos, Vietnam, Northwest China
	I2	ayw2	Laos, Vietnam
J		ayw	Japan

A ninth genotype (I) has recently been proposed after being found in north-western China [43], Eastern India [44], Laos [45] and Vietnam [45, 46]. Even more recently, a tentative new genotype "J" has been isolated in a single Japanese patient with HCC [47].

The two genotypes responsible for the majority of infections in Europe are genotype A (mainly subgenotype A2) in the north-western part of Europe and genotype D (mainly subgenotypes D1, D2 and D3) in the south-eastern Europe and the Mediterranean area [3].

The Origin of HBV

A number of conflicting hypotheses have been made concerning the origin of HBV. It has been proposed that it originated in the New World and spread to the rest of the world as a result of European colonisation over the last 400 years [48]. This conflicts with the observation of its widespread distribution among wild Old World apes (chimpanzees, orang-utans and gibbons). A second hypothesis proposes a co-divergence of HBV and its (human and non-human) primate hosts over a period of about 10–35 million years [49], but this implies a very slow evolutionary rate that is incompatible with current molecular clock estimates, indicating a faster rate of evolution [50–52]. Moreover, the viruses isolated from non-human primates show the same divergence as those observed among human genotypes, and their phylogenetic patterns show that the relationship between non-human viruses and some human genotypes is closer than that of other human genotypes, suggesting different viral leaps from primates to humans and vice versa and excluding the idea of virus/primate co-divergence [53]. A third hypothesis is that HBV was present in anatomically modern humans and spread as a result of their migrations over the last 100,000 years or so [54].

The main difficulty in reconstructing the HBV phylodynamics is the lack of a consensus in the estimation of the rate of evolution of the virus that also affects the tMRCA estimates and the timescales of HBV evolution [52].

Support for the hypothesis of the long co-evolution of HBV genotypes in humans comes from the two American genotypes F and H, which are inter-related and diverge significantly from the other HBV genotypes. As described above, we know that HBV-F subgenotypes are distributed in different areas and aboriginal tribes [55] in which the prevalence of infection is very high (up to 30 %) [56, 57]. This suggests that they have been generated by the evolution of the virus in small and isolated populations. On the basis of genetic studies, all aboriginal Americans came from a population originating in the region between the Altai and Amur that reached Beringia between 30 and 22 ky and North America 16.6 ky [58]. This founding population probably consisted of fewer than 5000 people [59] divided into bands of probably less than 100, who reached North America in successive waves over a period of 1500 years or more [60]. Moreover, the very high prevalence of HBV subgenotype C2 found in the small Jarawa tribe of the Andaman Islands that remained in complete isolation for thousands of years cannot plausibly be attributed to recent contact with the virus, despite the quite limited divergence from the sequences of the same subgenotype presently circulating in Thailand [61]. However, this apparent discrepancy may find an explanation taking as a reference the sequence belonging to the same genotype recently extracted from the liver cells of a Korean mummy dated 400–500 years ago [62], suggesting that the evolutionary rate of this genotype may be slower than previously expected.

In some of these small, numerically stable and isolated groups, HBV could easily have become hyper-endemic and prevalently transmitted vertically. The resulting immunological tolerance would have reduced the selective pressure of host immunity on the virus, thus justifying a slow evolutionary rate. Very different evolutionary rates have recently been demonstrated in subjects with and without serum HBeAg [63], and HBeAg positivity, associated with slower rates, is a prerequisite for efficient vertical transmission [64].

On the contrary, the penetration of HBV into large, fast-changing, highly mobile and susceptible populations depends on other, mainly horizontal, transmission routes, which may also be responsible for higher evolutionary rates. The rate of vertical transmission is relatively low in populations in which the prevalent HBV genotypes are those associated with high rates of HBeAg negativity (such as genotype D), and horizontal transmissions such as the parenteral (iatrogenic practices and intravenous drug use) and intra-familiar routes play a more important role [64]. The main circulation among immunocompetent HBeAg negative adults justifies a faster evolution of the virus because of stronger selective pressure. Moreover, HBV in these populations is generally characterised by high basic reproduction numbers (R_0) of 1–2 estimated in various ways [52, 65, 66], which indicates a very rapid spread of the virus in susceptible communities and once again conflicts with the hypothesis of a slow evolutionary rate.

The Origin and Evolution of Genotype D

The HBV genotype D is one of the two most prevalent genotypes in Europe, in particular in the north-eastern countries and in the Mediterranean basin, including northern Africa, and the Middle East. It is also highly prevalent on the Indian sub-continent and a group of islands in the Indian Ocean with high endemic levels of HBV [67], and has additionally been identified in Oceania [40]. Nine HBV-D subgenotypes (D1–D9) have so far been described (Fig. 2.1), showing a different geographic distribution. Subgenotype D1 is widespread in Greece, Turkey and north Africa [68, 69]; D2 in north-eastern Europe (Russia, Belarus, Estonia) and Albania [70, 71]; and D3 in Italy and Serbia [72, 73]. D4 is the dominant subgenotype in Oceania [40]; D5 in primitive tribes living in India, where a number of different D subgenotypes are also found [74]; D6 in Papua and Indonesia [75]; D7 in Tunisia and Morocco [76, 77]. Finally, the recently described D8 and D9 subgenotypes have been identified in Nigeria and India, and have been recognised as recombinant forms of genotype D with E [78] or C [79].

A number of preliminary studies agree about a relatively recent origin of genotype D in the early twentieth century [52, 80] in Europe, with two phases of expansion: the first in the 1940s and 1950s and the second occurring from the 1960s until the 1980s, when the growth of the genotype reached a plateau. It was hypothesised that the initial event underlying viral penetration in Europe were the two World Wars at that time when the use of unsafe medical injections was common and there was an increase in the use of blood and blood derivatives for transfusion purposes [81] before

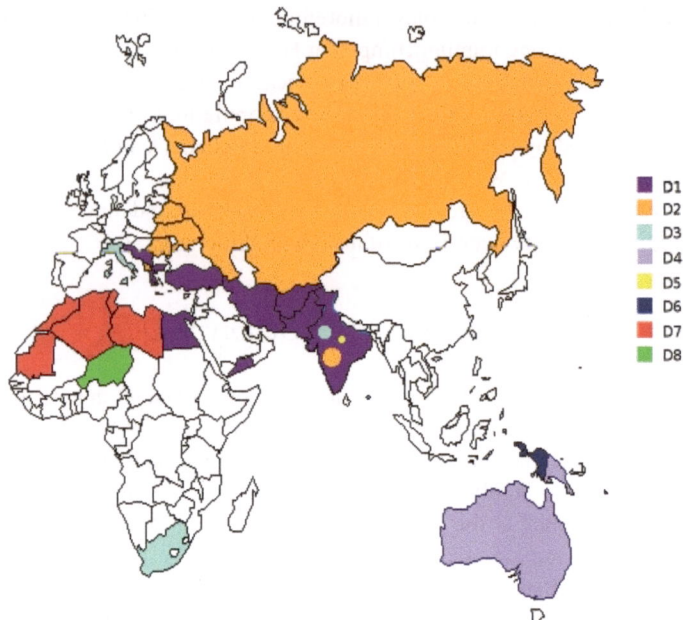

Fig. 2.1 Distribution of hepatitis B virus (HBV) subgenotypes D in Eurasia and the Mediterranean basin. Countries are coloured on the basis of their prevalent subgenotypes (see legend)

HBsAg screening became available in the 1970s [82]. Later, the further expansion was attributable to percutaneous transmission among intravenous drug users (IDUs) and other people exposed to infected blood. In particular, subgenotype HBV-D3 was shown to be associated with percutaneous transmission and drug addiction [72, 83]. The virus isolated from IVDUs is characterised by a number of S and P gene mutations [72], such as the main mutation in residue 125 (S125T) of S protein, which has been described by various authors all over the developed world [40, 52, 80, 84]. A plateau of the epidemic was reached in the 1980s, in relation to the decrease in acute HBV infections in developed countries [52, 85, 86].

A recent and comprehensive reconstruction of the epidemiological history of HBV genotype D obtained using a phylogeographical approach [87] indicates that it originated in the second half of the nineteenth century in India and that subgenotype D5 (an indigenous Indian subgenotype) was probably the first to diverge. The common ancestors left India and reached central Asia in the first decade of the twentieth century, when subgenotypes D1–D3 diverged. Subsequently (between the 1930s and 1940s), they spread to Europe and the Mediterranean area by means of at least two routes: a south-western route (mainly because of the diffusion of subgenotype D1) crossing the Middle East and reaching north Africa and the south-eastern Mediterranean; and a second north-western route (closely associated with D2) that crossed the former Soviet Union and reached eastern Europe and the Mediterranean through Albania [66].

This reconstruction makes it possible to hypothesise that the First and Second World Wars played a crucial role in the global spread of HBV-D from India to the rest of the world, but the further spread of the infection (particularly in south-eastern Europe, the Middle East and northern Africa) was probably sustained by the unsafe use of injections in medical practice. Events such as outbreaks of jaundice following the intravenous injection of arsphenamine (for anti-syphilis treatment) from the early 1920s to the late 1940s, led to the spread of some HBV-D subgenotypes to Europe [88].

In the populations in which HBV-D predominates (which are characterised by a high rate of mutations causing HBeAg negativity), the majority of infections are acquired horizontally, mainly as a result of household contacts or because of the use of unsterilised needles and syringes [89, 90].

The Origin and Evolution of Genotype A

Genotype A is an ubiquitous genotype, largely spread over four continents: Africa, Europe, Asia and America. It has been classified into seven distinct evolutionary groups. Subgenotype A1 is highly prevalent in southern and east Africa (South Africa, Uganda, Malawi, Tanzania, Congo, Somalia) and south Asia (India, the Philippines, Bangladesh, Nepal) [40, 74, 91–93]. Subgenotype A2 is the most widespread in Europe and North America [40, 91] and has also been isolated in South Africa [94]. It has been suggested that genotype A might have originated in Africa and hypothesised the importation of HBV-A2 from Africa to Europe by Portuguese sailors in the sixteenth and seventeenth centuries, and the arrival of A1 in Asia as a consequence of trade and travel between eastern Africa and southern Asia [95]. The more recently described subgenotypes are A3 in Pygmies and Bantus living in Cameroon and Gabon [96, 97]; a "tentative A4" from Mali; and a subgenotype A5 isolated in patients from Nigeria (Fig. 2.2) [98]. Interestingly, HBV-A5 has also been found in Haiti, which suggests that it might have been the dominant subgenotype in an area near the current Nigeria (formerly the Bight of Benin) before the time of the slave trade (between the eighteenth and nineteenth centuries). An HBV-A6 has only been reported in African–Belgian patients [84] and a new "tentative subgenotype A7" has been isolated in Cameroon [99]. It has recently been proposed to classify A3, "tentative A4", A5 and "tentative A7" within a single subgenotype called "quasi subgenotype A3", because they share a common ancestor, but none of them meets the criterion necessary for the definition of "subgenotype" (a genetic divergence of 4–8%) [84] and a new classification, consisting of three subgenotypes (A1, A2 and A4-formerly subgenotype A6) and one West-African quasi-subgenotype (A3) has been proposed [100].

Subgenotype A2 is the most prevalent genotype in the developed countries, in particular in the USA and north-west Europe, and in the last few years its prevalence has also been growing in Japan [101]. Several studies have demonstrated a relatively recent penetration of HBV-A in Europe, between the 1960s and 1980s and an association of this subgenotype with people acquiring the infection as a result of sexual transmission, particularly men-having-sex-with-men (MSM) [52, 102].

A single clonal strain has been isolated among high-risk subjects all over the world [2, 103], suggesting a relatively recent distinct worldwide HBV-A2 epidemic among MSM, now also spreading among heterosexuals [103].

It seems that the epidemiological dichotomy of Europe (which makes genotype D the most prevalent genotype in eastern and southern Europe, where HBV is highly endemic, and genotype A the main strain in central and northern Europe, where HBV is less widespread) could be due to the differences in their main routes of transmission, as has been observed in Italy [52]: predominantly parenteral transmission in highly endemic areas (unsafe injections, intra-family transmission), and hetero- and homosexual transmission in less endemic areas [2, 90, 102].

In contrast, HBV-A1 probably originated in Africa and the slave trade and colonisation played a major role in its global dispersion: in particular, the Arabian East African slave trade from Africa to India (until the late nineteenth century), the Belgian colonisation of the Congo (in the first half of the twentieth century), and the European slave trade (until the nineteenth century) [104].

The Origin and Evolution of Genotype E

Genotype E is the most prevalent strain of HBV in central and western Africa (see Fig. 2.2) [105]. It has a very low degree of genetic diversity: the isolates obtained so far form a single monophyletic group [106]. The absence of any significant spread among

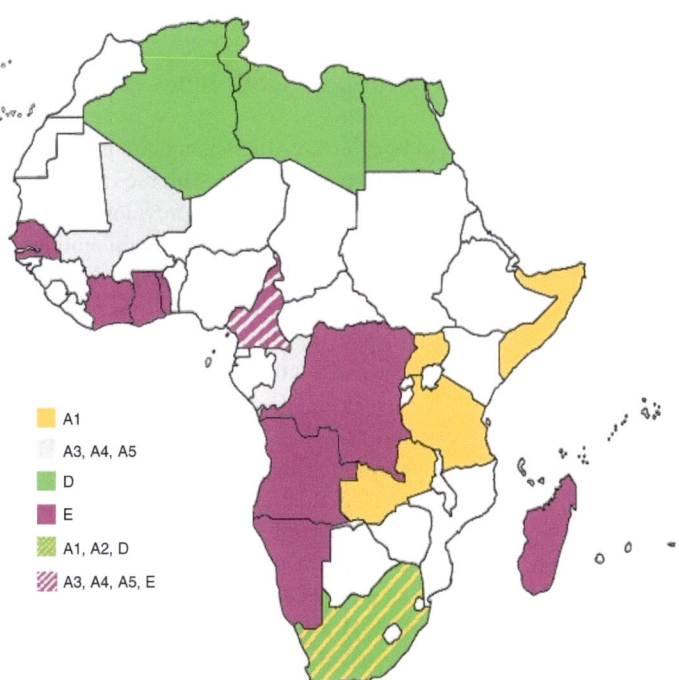

Fig. 2.2 Distribution of HBV genotypes in Africa. Countries are coloured on the basis of their prevalent geno-/subgenotypes (see legend)

Afro-Americans, despite the forced immigration of western African slaves [106], indicates that it was probably rare in west Africa at the time of the slave trade and before the nineteenth century. The high prevalence and low degree of genetic divergence of HBV-E suggest its recent explosive spread in west Africa after the end of the slave trade approximately 200 years ago [107]. Recent estimates suggest a penetration of HBV-E in Central West Africa around 60 years ago with an exponential growth of the epidemic between 30 and 40 years ago. These observations support the view that the explosive spread of HBV-E in Africa must have been due to a new and highly efficient route of transmission, probably the unsafe use of needles during numerous mass-vaccination campaigns (against yaws, sleeping sickness, smallpox and measles), which were particularly frequent in west/central Africa between the 1920s and 1960s [107, 108]. In this way, HBV-E brought to the substitution of other, endemic genotypes such as HBV-A5.

The Origin and Evolution of Genotypes F and H

Genotypes F and H are indigenous to America and the most prevalent HBV genotypes in central/south America with the exception of the Afro-Brazilian community, where the most prevalent subgenotype is A1 [109]. Genotype F is the predominant strain among the Amerindians of the Amazon basin [110]. It is classified into four subgenotypes (F1–F4), and further sub-divided into different clades. As shown in Fig. 2.3, F1 is highly prevalent in central America (clade F1a), Alaska and south-east America (clade F1b) [111, 112]; F2 is highly prevalent in Venezuela (clades F2a and b) and is also present in Brazil (clade F2a alone) [111]; F3 is present in central (Panama) and northern Latin America (Colombia and Venezuela); and F4 is present in Bolivia and Argentina (where it co-circulates with F1b) [113]. Genotype H is predominant in Mexico, where it represents more than 50% of infections, even in some native Mexican populations [114], thus suggesting an ancient origin (pre-Hispanic) of HBV-H in the Aztec population. From a phylogenetic point of view, genotypes F and H share a common ancestor and are highly divergent from Old World HBV genotypes

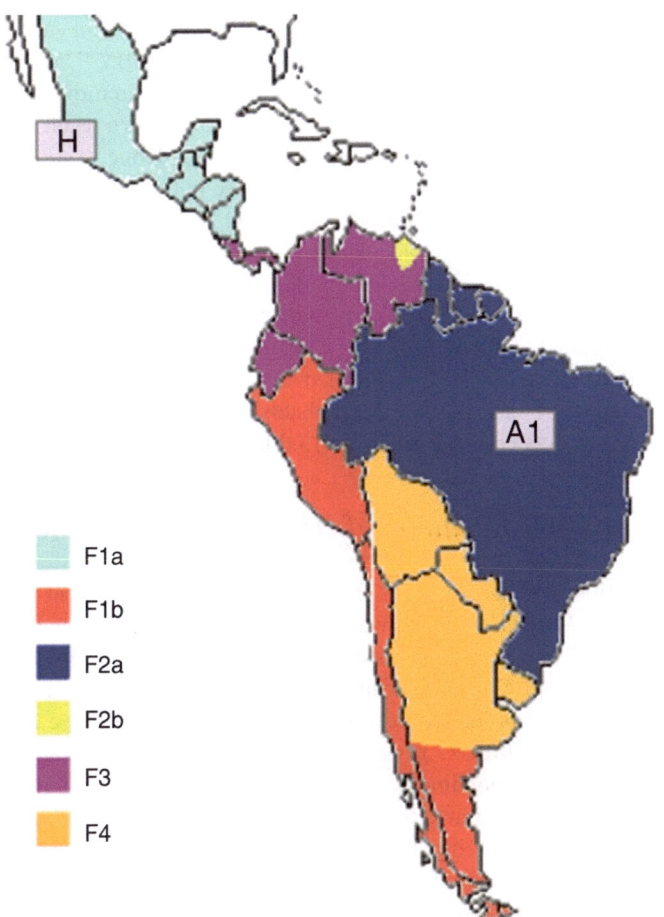

Fig. 2.3 Distribution of HBV F subgenotypes in Latin America. Countries are coloured on the basis of their prevalent geno-/subgenotypes (see legend)

[42], being closer to an isolate obtained from a New World monkey (the woolly monkey). These data suggest that genotypes F and H might have split off a long time ago, and possibly represent the result of a cross-species transfer [42].

The estimation of the phylogeography of HBV-F on a calendar time scale suggested the pre-Columbian origin of HBV-F and their subgenotypes, some of which would have disappeared during the conquests of the sixteenth and seventeenth century as a result of the extreme decline in population numbers. The epidemic would have then expanded because of the rapid increase in the Latin American population since the eighteenth century [113].

A study of the molecular epidemiology and evolutionary dynamics of HBV-F in Colombia demonstrated that HBV-F3 was probably the oldest F subgenotype originating in Venezuela and is most related to genotype H [111].

Recent studies [115] estimated an origin of the Amerindian genotypes (F and H), which probably followed the initial New World settlers coming from Asia 13,000 years ago.

Origin and Evolution of HBV Genotypes B and C

Hepatitis B virus genotypes B and C are the most prevalent geno-types in Asia. Genotype B was identified in 2002 and immediately classified into two subgenotypes: Bj, largely spread in Japan and Ba, present in Asia, but not in Japan. Subgenotype Ba was demon-strated to be a product of recombination between a genotype B and a genotype C PreC/C gene. In 2004, it was proposed to rename them B1 (corresponding to the former Bj) and B2 (former Ba) [40]. Genotype B is characterised by a large spread in Asian and Arctic populations and is highly heterogeneous: nine different subgeno-types have been identified so far. Some of them are recombinant: subgenotype B2, subgenotypes B3 (isolated in Indonesia), B4 (identified in Vietnam) and B5 (identified in the Philippines). Another non-recombinant subgenotype was B6, identified in an indigenous Arctic population and in southwestern China in the Yunnan region. Subgenotypes B7, B8 and B9 were all identified on different islands of Indonesia suggesting a correlation between the B subgenotype and the ethnicity of the infected patients [116].

Genotype C shows the highest level of genetic heterogeneity, being classified into at least 16 different subgenotypes, which dis-play different ethnogeographic distribution. Subgenotypes C1 and C2 (initially named Cs and Ce) are the most widely distributed subgenotypes in Southeast Asia (Vietnam, Myanmar, Southern China, Thailand) and the Far East (Korea, Japan, Northern China) respectively. Subgenotype C4 is found in the aboriginal population of Australia, while all the other subgenotypes are present in the Philippines and Indonesia [116].

On the basis of a recent study, HBV genotype C could be the oldest human genotype, originating about 30.0 ky ago [54]. Accordingly, a recent study detected HBV nucleic acids in a Korean mummy of the sixteenth century, which was clustered with subgenotype C2 [62]. The concordance between the HBV subgenotype and geographic localisation and the great similarity of this strain to the C2 isolates presently circulating [62] suggest a relatively low rate of evolution of HBV, at least of genotype C.

Other Geno-/Subgenotypes of Interest

Genotype G was found in several European countries, in the USA, in Japan and in Mexico [117]. All known isolates have both PreC/C and BCP mutations, preventing the ability of this genotype to give (alone) chronic infections. For this reason, in chronically infected patients, genotype G is always in coinfection with another genotype that can supply the HBeAg [118]. An association between HBV genotype G and sexual transmission, in particular among MSM, has been observed [119], thus justifying the frequent coinfection with subgenotype A2.

Clinical Implications of HBV Variability

HBeAg Expression and Viral Genotypes

The substitution of the G in position 1896 of the PreC/C gene with an A genotype abrogates the expression of HBeAg. Site 1896 is inserted into a stem-loop fundamental as an encapsidation signal, and is paired with the nucleotide in position 1858, which is a C in genotype A, but is a T in several other genotypes. The presence of a T in position 1858 makes the mutation (G to A) in position 1896 more stable. For this reason, several genotypes such as D, E, G and some B and C subgenotypes are more frequently subjected to preC/C mutation. In contrast, BCP mutations are more prominent in HBV genotypes A, F and the other HBV B and C subgenotypes. These data suggest that subjects infected by some HBV genotypes (D, E, G) are more likely to be affected by HBeAg-negative chronic hepatitis [120].

In general, Asian subjects have a longer persistence of HBeAg positivity in their blood. The anti-HBe seroconversion occurs earlier and more frequently in subjects infected with genotype B than in those with genotype C [121]. A possible hypothesis is that genotype B HBV might develop the G1896A mutation, which abolishes the e antigen expression, while genotype C develops BCP mutations that reduce but do not abolish HBeAg expression [120].

In Western Europe, where the predominant genotypes are D and A2, the rate of sustained remission after HBeAg seroconversion is higher in genotype A than in genotype D [120]. Even in this case, the reason may be the higher frequency of PreC/C mutations inducing the reactivation of the viral replication in genotype D than in genotype A, as also suggested by the higher prevalence of HBeAg positivity in the latter [120, 122].

Progression of the Infection

Cirrhosis and HCC are the most significant complications of chronic hepatitis B (CHB). Given that the viral genotype may influence the natural history of the infection and that viral genotypes are differently distributed throughout the world, the pattern of the development of complications also varies on a geographical basis.

Several studies have suggested that the risk of cirrhosis development in Europe (where genotypes A and D are prevalent) might be higher than in East Asia, where the most prevalent genotypes are B and C, C2 (mean incidence rate of 6.75 vs 2.2 per 100 person-years respectively) [120]. This difference is in part due to the higher incidence of genotype D infection, associated with HBeAg-negative CHB, in Europe than in East Asia.

Accumulating evidence indicated that higher plasma HBV DNA levels, infection with HBV genotype C, in addition to mutations at 1653T, 1753V and A1762T/G1764A are independently associated with the risk of HCC in Asian men. This explains the correlation between HCC development and genotype C rather than genotype B (OR = 1.68 > 2.35 < 3.30) [123]. HBV genotype A1 in Africa is associated with a 4.5-fold increase in the relative risk of developing HCC compared with other genotypes [124].

HBV Genotype and CH Therapy

Several studies have indicated that the loss of HBeAg and anti-HBe seroconversion during interferon treatment are observed more frequently in patients with genotype A than in those with genotype D and, to a lesser degree, in patients with genotype B versus genotype C. In contrast, response rates to nucleoside/tide analogues are similar in the different genotypes. However, a different pattern of resistance-associated mutation may prevail [120] given that mutations at the polymerase coding gene may influence the appearance of mutations in the overlapping surface antigen. For example, the lamivudine and adefovir resistance mutation at position rt181 (from A to T) results in a stop codon in the overlapping surface antigen gene (in position 172). This variant has been associated with enhancing progression to HCC and is more prevalent in Asian patients with genotypes B and C than in European and North American patients with genotypes A and D [125].

Modes of Transmission

As mentioned before, different genotypes are dispersed within populations by different main routes of transmission. In particular, genotypes B and C, which are predominant in populations with a high level of endemicity, vertical/perinatal transmission is the prevalent mode of propagation. On the contrary, in the developed countries, where genotypes A2 and D prevail and the endemicity level is lower/intermediate, the main transmission routes are horizontal and highly efficient, and are sexual (associated with A2) and percutaneous (associated with genotype D). These differences may explain different characteristics in the natural history of infection due to HBV genotypes. For example, the longer persistence of the period of immunotolerance in HBV genotypes B and C may be useful in increasing the probability of transmission from the mother to the children. A HBeAg-positive mother has a probability of virtually 100% of transmitting the infection to an infant, who has a 90% risk of developing a chronic infection characterised by a long immune tolerant phase lasting decades, in which HBeAg positivity persists. Similarly, where intrafamilial or percutaneous (through unsafe injections or transfusions) transmission prevails (such as in the Mediterranean area and Africa), genotypes able to give long-lasting HBeAg-negative chronic infections characterised by intermittent flares and remissions, such as genotype D in the Mediterranean area or E in Western and Central Africa, could be selected [64].

The selective action of the prevalent mode of transmission at a population level on the different behavioural characteristics of the genotypes is well described by the differences between two closely related subgenotypes: HBV-A1 and -A2. In fact, subgenotype A1 is highly prevalent: the main mode of transmission at the population level is in the early childhood, whereas HBV-A2 is mainly transmitted through high-risk sexual contact [126]. In Africa, where the prevalence of infection is high, the transmission can easily occur through massive environmental contamination; in this condition, a self-limiting, HBeAg-positive infection is sufficient to infect cohabiting susceptible children. On the contrary, the main sexual transmission of genotype A2 in developed countries may explain its relative initial benignity and the higher rate of chronic infections mainly due to BCP mutations, reducing but not abrogating the HBeAg expression. Similar considerations can be made for genotype F, the most prevalent genotype in South America. This genotype is transmitted in early childhood on a community basis (rather than based on an individual family). Under these conditions, efficient transmission requires a highly dense and close population with a high level of HBV endemicity, to have sufficient numbers of HBeAg-positive transmitters. These conditions are met in Amerindian populations [126].

This observation may account for the common characteristics of genotypes F and A1 natural history as suggested by the high frequency of HCC [124, 127] and the frequent association with HBeAg-positive infection in both cases [128].

References

1. Ott JJ, Stevens GA, Groeger J, Wiersma ST. Global epidemiology of hepatitis B virus infection: new estimates of age-specific HBsAg seroprevalence and endemicity. Vaccine. 2012;30(12): 2212–9. doi:10.1016/j.vaccine.2011.12.116.

2. Rantala M, van de Laar MJ. Surveillance and epidemiology of hepatitis B and C in Europe—a review. Euro Surveill. 2008;13(21).

3. Schaefer S. Hepatitis B virus genotypes in Europe. Hepatol Res. 2007;37(s1):S20–6. doi:10.1111/j.1872-034X.2007.00099.x.

4. He B, Fan Q, Yang F, Hu T, Qiu W, Feng Y, Li Z, Li Y, Zhang F, Guo H, Zou X, Tu C. Hepatitis virus in long-fingered bats, Myanmar. Emerg Infect Dis. 2013;19(4):638–40. doi:10.3201/eid1904.121655.

5. Prince AM, Ikram H, Hopp TP. Hepatitis B virus vaccine: identification of HBsAg/a and HBsAg/d but not HBsAg/y subtype antigenic determinants on a synthetic immunogenic peptide. Proc Natl Acad Sci U S A. 1982;79(2):579–82.

6. Zoulim F, Saputelli J, Seeger C. Woodchuck hepatitis virus X protein is required for viral infection in vivo. J Virol. 1994;68(3):2026–30.

7. Tian Y, Yang W, Song J, Wu Y, Ni B. Hepatitis B virus X protein-induced aberrant epigenetic modifications contributing to human hepatocellular carcinoma pathogenesis. Mol Cell Biol. 2013;33(15):2810–6. doi:10.1128/mcb.00205-13.

8. Zoulim F. New insight on hepatitis B virus persistence from the study of intrahepatic viral cccDNA. J Hepatol. 2005;42(3):302–8. doi:10.1016/j.jhep.2004.12.015.

9. Mizokami M, Orito E, Ohba K, Ikeo K, Lau JY, Gojobori T. Constrained evolution with respect to gene overlap of hepatitis B virus. J Mol Evol. 1997;44 Suppl 1:S83–90.

10. Deny P, Zoulim F. Hepatitis B virus: from diagnosis to treatment. Pathol Biol. 2010;58(4):245–53. doi:10.1016/j.patbio.2010.05.002.

11. Harrison TJ. Hepatitis B virus: molecular virology and common mutants. Semin Liver Dis. 2006;26(2):87–96. doi:10.1055/s-2006-939754.

12. Locarnini S. Molecular virology of hepatitis B virus. Semin Liver Dis. 2004;24 Suppl 1:3–10. doi:10.1055/s-2004-828672.

13. Carman WF, Jacyna MR, Hadziyannis S, Karayiannis P, McGarvey MJ, Makris A, Thomas HC. Mutation preventing formation of hepatitis B e antigen in patients with chronic hepatitis B infection. Lancet. 1989;2(8663):588–91.

14. Laskus T, Rakela J, Nowicki MJ, Persing DH. Hepatitis B virus core promoter sequence analysis in fulminant and chronic hepatitis B. Gastroenterology. 1995;109(5):1618–23.

15. Liang TJ, Hasegawa K, Rimon N, Wands JR, Ben-Porath E. A hepatitis B virus mutant associated with an epidemic of fulminant hepatitis. N Engl J Med. 1991;324(24):1705–9. doi:10.1056/nejm199106133242405.

16. Omata M, Ehata T, Yokosuka O, Hosoda K, Ohto M. Mutations in the precore region of hepatitis B virus DNA in patients with fulminant and severe hepatitis. N Engl J Med. 1991;324(24):1699–704. doi:10.1056/nejm199106133242404.

17. Laskus T, Persing DH, Nowicki MJ, Mosley JW, Rakela J. Nucleotide sequence analysis of the precore region in patients with fulminant hepatitis B in the United States. Gastroenterology. 1993;105(4): 1173–8.

18. Liang TJ, Hasegawa K, Munoz SJ, Shapiro CN, Yoffe B, McMahon BJ, Feng C, Bei H, Alter MJ, Dienstag JL. Hepatitis B virus precore mutation and fulminant hepatitis in the United States. A polymerase chain reaction-based assay for the detection of specific mutation. J Clin Invest. 1994;93(2):550–5. doi:10.1172/jci117006.

19. Blum HE, Galun E, Liang TJ, von Weizsacker F, Wands JR. Naturally occurring missense mutation in the polymerase gene terminating hepatitis B virus replication. J Virol. 1991;65(4):1836–42.

20. Liaw YF, Chu CM. Hepatitis B virus infection. Lancet. 2009;373(9663):582–92. doi:10.1016/s0140-6736(09)60207-5.

21. Allen MI, Deslauriers M, Andrews CW, Tipples GA, Walters KA, Tyrrell DL, Brown N, Condreay LD. Identification and characterization of mutations in hepatitis B virus resistant to lamivudine. Lamivudine Clinical Investigation Group. Hepatology. 1998;27(6):1670–7. doi:10.1002/hep.510270628.

22. Locarnini SA, Yuen L. Molecular genesis of drug-resistant and vaccine-escape HBV mutants. Antivir Ther. 2010;15(3 Pt B):451–61. doi:10.3851/imp1499.

23. Torresi J. The virological and clinical significance of mutations in the overlapping envelope and polymerase genes of hepatitis B virus. J Clin Virol. 2002;25(2):97–106.

24. Raimondo G, Costantino L, Caccamo G, Pollicino T, Squadrito G, Cacciola I, Brancatelli S. Non-sequencing molecular approaches to identify preS2-defective hepatitis B virus variants proved to be associated with severe liver diseases. J Hepatol. 2004;40(3):515–9. doi:10.1016/j.jhep.2003.11.025.

25. Zanetti AR, Tanzi E, Manzillo G, Maio G, Sbreglia C, Caporaso N, Thomas H, Zuckerman AJ. Hepatitis B variant in Europe. Lancet. 1988;2(8620):1132–3.

26. Ogata N, Zanetti AR, Yu M, Miller RH, Purcell RH. Infectivity and pathogenicity in chimpanzees of a surface gene mutant of hepatitis B virus that emerged in a vaccinated infant. J Infect Dis. 1997;175(3):511–23.

27. Coleman PF, Chen YC, Mushahwar IK. Immunoassay detection of hepatitis B surface antigen mutants. J Med Virol. 1999;59(1):19–24.

28. Mimms L. Hepatitis B virus escape mutants: "pushing the envelope" of chronic hepatitis B virus infection. Hepatology. 1995;21(3):884–7.

29. Carman WF, Zanetti AR, Karayiannis P, Waters J, Manzillo G, Tanzi E, Zuckerman AJ, Thomas HC. Vaccine-induced escape mutant of hepatitis B virus. Lancet. 1990;336(8711):325–9.

30. Harrison TJ, Hopes EA, Oon CJ, Zanetti AR, Zuckerman AJ. Independent emergence of a vaccine-induced escape mutant of hepatitis B virus. J Hepatol. 1991;13 Suppl 4:S105–7.

31. Hsu HY, Chang MH, Ni YH, Lin HH, Wang SM, Chen DS. Surface gene mutants of hepatitis B virus in infants who develop acute or chronic infections despite immunoprophylaxis. Hepatology. 1997;26(3):786–91. doi:10.1002/hep.510260336.

32. Zuckerman AJ, Harrison TJ, Oon CJ. Mutations in S region of hepatitis B virus. Lancet. 1994;343(8899):737–8.

33. Fortuin M, Karthigesu V, Allison L, Howard C, Hoare S, Mendy M, Whittle HC. Breakthrough infections and identification of a viral variant in Gambian children immunized with hepatitis B vaccine. J Infect Dis. 1994;169(6):1374–6.

34. Terrault NA, Zhou S, McCory RW, Pruett TL, Lake JR, Roberts JP, Ascher NL, Wright TL. Incidence and clinical consequences of surface and polymerase gene mutations in liver transplant recipients on hepatitis B immunoglobulin. Hepatology. 1998;28(2):555–61. doi:10.1002/hep.510280237.

35. Basuni AA, Butterworth L, Cooksley G, Locarnini S, Carman WF. Prevalence of HBsAg mutants and impact of hepatitis B infant immunisation in four Pacific Island countries. Vaccine. 2004;22(21–22):2791–9. doi:10.1016/j.vaccine.2004.01.046.

36. Ogata N, Cote PJ, Zanetti AR, Miller RH, Shapiro M, Gerin J, Purcell RH. Licensed recombinant hepatitis B vaccines protect chimpanzees against infection with the prototype surface gene mutant of hepatitis B virus. Hepatology. 1999;30(3):779–86. doi:10.1002/hep.510300309.

37. Purcell RH. Hepatitis B virus mutants and efficacy of vaccination. Lancet. 2000;356(9231):769–70. doi:10.1016/s0140-6736(05)73670-9.

38. Mele A, Tancredi F, Romano L, Giuseppone A, Colucci M, Sangiuolo A, Lecce R, Adamo B, Tosti ME, Taliani G, Zanetti AR. Effectiveness of hepatitis B vaccination in babies born to hepatitis B surface antigen-positive mothers in Italy. J Infect Dis. 2001;184(7):905–8. doi:10.1086/323396.

39. El Chaar M, Candotti D, Crowther RA, Allain JP. Impact of hepatitis B virus surface protein mutations on the diagnosis of occult hepatitis B virus infection. Hepatology. 2010;52(5):1600–10. doi:10.1002/hep.23886.

40. Norder H, Courouce AM, Coursaget P, Echevarria JM, Lee SD, Mushahwar IK, Robertson BH, Locarnini S, Magnius LO. Genetic diversity of hepatitis B virus strains derived worldwide: genotypes, subgenotypes, and HBsAg subtypes. Intervirology. 2004;47(6):289–309. doi:10.1159/000080872.

41. Stuyver L, De Gendt S, Van Geyt C, Zoulim F, Fried M, Schinazi RF, Rossau R. A new genotype of hepatitis B virus: complete genome and phylogenetic relatedness. J Gen Virol. 2000;81(Pt 1):67–74.

42. Arauz-Ruiz P, Norder H, Robertson BH, Magnius LO. Genotype H: a new Amerindian genotype of hepatitis B virus revealed in Central America. J Gen Virol. 2002;83(Pt 8):2059–73.

43. Yu H, Yuan Q, Ge SX, Wang HY, Zhang YL, Chen QR, Zhang J, Chen PJ, Xia NS. Molecular and phylogenetic analyses suggest an additional hepatitis B virus genotype "I". PLoS One. 2010;5(2):e9297. doi:10.1371/journal.pone.0009297.

44. Arankalle VA, Gandhe SS, Borkakoty BJ, Walimbe AM, Biswas D, Mahanta J. A novel HBV recombinant (genotype I) similar to Vietnam/Laos in a primitive tribe in eastern India. J Viral Hepat. 2010;17(7):501–10. doi:10.1111/j.1365-2893.2009.01206.x.

45. Olinger CM, Jutavijittum P, Hubschen JM, Yousukh A, Samountry B, Thammavong T, Toriyama K, Muller CP. Possible new hepatitis B virus genotype, southeast Asia. Emerg Infect Dis. 2008;14(11):1777–80. doi:10.3201/eid1411.080437.

46. Tran TT, Trinh TN, Abe K. New complex recombinant genotype of hepatitis B virus identified in Vietnam. J Virol. 2008;82(11):5657–63. doi:10.1128/jvi.02556-07.

47. Tatematsu K, Tanaka Y, Kurbanov F, Sugauchi F, Mano S, Maeshiro T, Nakayoshi T, Wakuta M, Miyakawa Y, Mizokami M. A genetic variant of hepatitis B virus divergent from known human and ape genotypes isolated from a Japanese patient and provisionally assigned to new genotype J. J Virol. 2009;83(20):10538–47. doi:10.1128/jvi.00462-09.

48. Bollyky P, Rambaut A, Grassly N, Carman W, Holmes E. Hepatitis B virus has a recent new world evolutionary origin. Hepatology. 1997;4:765. WB Saunders Co., Independence Square West Curtis Center, Ste 300, Philadelphia, PA 19106-3399.

49. MacDonald DM, Holmes EC, Lewis JC, Simmonds P. Detection of hepatitis B virus infection in wild-born chimpanzees (Pan troglodytes verus): phylogenetic relationships with human and other primate genotypes. J Virol. 2000;74(9):4253–7.

50. Fares MA, Holmes EC. A revised evolutionary history of hepatitis B virus (HBV). J Mol Evol. 2002;54(6):807–14. doi:10.1007/s00239-001-0084-z.

51. Orito E, Mizokami M, Ina Y, Moriyama EN, Kameshima N, Yamamoto M, Gojobori T. Host-independent evolution and a genetic classification of the hepadnavirus family based on nucleotide sequences. Proc Natl Acad Sci U S A. 1989;86(18):7059–62.

52. Zehender G, De Maddalena C, Giambelli C, Milazzo L, Schiavini M, Bruno R, Tanzi E, Galli M. Different evolutionary rates and epidemic growth of hepatitis B virus genotypes A and D. Virology. 2008;380(1):84–90. doi:10.1016/j.virol.2008.07.009.

53. Holmes EC. Evolutionary history and phylogeography of human viruses. Annu Rev Microbiol. 2008;62:307–28. doi:10.1146/annurev.micro.62.081307.162912.

54. Paraskevis D, Magiorkinis G, Magiorkinis E, Ho SY, Belshaw R, Allain JP, Hatzakis A. Dating the origin and dispersal of hepatitis B virus infection in humans and primates. Hepatology. 2013;57(3):908–16. doi:10.1002/hep.26079.

55. Devesa M, Pujol FH. Hepatitis B virus genetic diversity in Latin America. Virus Res. 2007;127(2):177–84. doi:10.1016/j.virusres.2007.01.004.

56. Braga WS. [Hepatitis B and D virus infection within Amerindians ethnic groups in the Brazilian Amazon: epidemiological aspects]. Rev Soc Bras Med Trop. 2004;37 Suppl 2:9–13.

57. Echevarria JM, Leon P. Epidemiology of viruses causing chronic hepatitis among populations from the Amazon Basin and related ecosystems. Cad Saude Publica. 2003;19(6):1583–91.

58. Tamm E, Kivisild T, Reidla M, Metspalu M, Smith DG, Mulligan CJ, Bravi CM, Rickards O, Martinez-Labarga C, Khusnutdinova EK, Fedorova SA, Golubenko MV, Stepanov VA, Gubina MA, Zhadanov SI, Ossipova LP, Damba L, Voevoda MI, Dipierri JE, Villems R, Malhi RS. Beringian standstill and spread of Native American founders. PLoS One. 2007;2(9):e829. doi:10.1371/journal.pone.0000829.

59. Kitchen A, Miyamoto MM, Mulligan CJ. A three-stage colonization model for the peopling of the Americas. PLoS One. 2008;3(2):e1596. doi:10.1371/journal.pone.0001596.

60. Goebel T, Waters MR, O'Rourke DH. The late Pleistocene dispersal of modern humans in the Americas. Science. 2008;319(5869):1497–502. doi:10.1126/science.1153569.

61. Murhekar MV, Chakravarty R, Murhekar KM, Banerjee A, Sehgal SC. Hepatitis B virus genotypes among the Jarawas: a primitive Negrito tribe of Andaman and Nicobar Islands, India. Arch Virol. 2006;151(8):1499–510. doi:10.1007/s00705-006-0737-8.

62. Kahila Bar-Gal G, Kim MJ, Klein A, Shin DH, Oh CS, Kim JW, Kim TH, Kim SB, Grant PR, Pappo O, Spigelman M, Shouval D. Tracing hepatitis B virus to the 16th century in a Korean mummy. Hepatology. 2012;56(5):1671–80. doi:10.1002/hep.25852.

63. Harrison A, Lemey P, Hurles M, Moyes C, Horn S, Pryor J, Malani J, Supuri M, Masta A, Teriboriki B, Toatu T, Penny D, Rambaut A, Shapiro B. Genomic analysis of hepatitis B virus reveals antigen state and genotype as sources of evolutionary rate variation. Viruses. 2011;3(2):83–101. doi:10.3390/v3020083.

64. Hadziyannis SJ. Natural history of chronic hepatitis B in Euro-Mediterranean and African countries. J Hepatol. 2011;55(1):183–91. doi:10.1016/j.jhep.2010.12.030.

65. Kretzschmar M, de Wit GA, Smits LJ, van de Laar MJ. Vaccination against hepatitis B in low endemic countries. Epidemiol Infect. 2002;128(2):229–44.

66. Zehender G, Shkjezi R, Ebranati E, Gabanelli E, Abazaj Z, Tanzi E, Kraja D, Bino S, Ciccozzi M, Galli M. Reconstruction of the epidemic history of hepatitis B virus genotype D in Albania. Infect Genet Evol. 2012;12(2):291–8. doi:10.1016/j.meegid.2011.11.009.

67. Murhekar MV, Murhekar KM, Sehgal SC. Epidemiology of hepatitis B virus infection among the tribes of Andaman and Nicobar Islands, India. Trans R Soc Trop Med Hyg. 2008;102(8):729–34. doi:10.1016/j.trstmh.2008.04.044.

68. Bozdayi G, Turkyilmaz AR, Idilman R, Karatayli E, Rota S, Yurdaydin C, Bozdayi AM. Complete genome sequence and phylogenetic analysis of hepatitis B virus isolated from Turkish patients with chronic HBV infection. J Med Virol. 2005;76(4):476–81. doi:10.1002/jmv.20386.

69. Garmiri P, Rezvan H, Abolghasemi H, Allain JP. Full genome characterization of hepatitis B virus strains from blood donors in Iran. J Med Virol. 2011;83(6):948–52. doi:10.1002/jmv.21772.

70. Tallo T, Tefanova V, Priimagi L, Schmidt J, Katargina O, Michailov M, Mukomolov S, Magnius L, Norder H. D2: major subgenotype of hepatitis B virus in Russia and the Baltic region. J Gen Virol. 2008;89(Pt 8):1829–39. doi:10.1099/vir.0.83660-0.

71. Zehender G, Ebranati E, Bernini F, Lo Presti A, Rezza G, Delogu M, Galli M, Ciccozzi M. Phylogeography and epidemiological history of West Nile virus genotype 1a in Europe and the Mediterranean basin. Infect Genet Evol. 2011;11(3):646–53. doi:10.1016/j.meegid.2011.02.003.

72. De Maddalena C, Giambelli C, Tanzi E, Colzani D, Schiavini M, Milazzo L, Bernini F, Ebranati E, Cargnel A, Bruno R, Galli M, Zehender G. High level of genetic heterogeneity in S and P genes of genotype D hepatitis B virus. Virology. 2007;365(1):113–24. doi:10.1016/j.virol.2007.03.015.

73. Lazarevic I, Cupic M, Delic D, Svirtlih NS, Simonovic J, Jovanovic T. Distribution of HBV genotypes, subgenotypes and HBsAg subtypes among chronically infected patients in Serbia. Arch Virol. 2007;152(11):2017–25. doi:10.1007/s00705-007-1031-0.

74. Banerjee A, Kurbanov F, Datta S, Chandra PK, Tanaka Y, Mizokami M, Chakravarty R. Phylogenetic relatedness and genetic diversity of hepatitis B virus isolates in Eastern India. J Med Virol. 2006;78(9):1164–74. doi:10.1002/jmv.20677.

75. Lusida MI, Nugrahaputra VE, Soetjipto, Handajani R, Nagano-Fujii M, Sasayama M, Utsumi T, Hotta H (2008) Novel subgenotypes of hepatitis B virus genotypes C and D in Papua, Indonesia. J Clin Microbiol. 46(7):2160–6. doi:10.1128/jcm.01681-07.

76. Kitab B, El Feydi AE, Afifi R, Derdabi O, Cherradi Y, Benazzouz M, Rebbani K, Brahim I, Salih Alj H, Zoulim F, Trepo C, Chemin I, Ezzikouri S, Benjelloun S. Hepatitis B genotypes/subgenotypes and MHR variants among Moroccan chronic carriers. J Infect. 2011;63(1):66–75. doi:10.1016/j.jinf.2011.05.007.

77. Meldal BH, Moula NM, Barnes IH, Boukef K, Allain JP. A novel hepatitis B virus subgenotype, D7, in Tunisian blood donors. J Gen Virol. 2009;90(Pt 7):1622–8. doi:10.1099/vir.0.009738-0.

78. Abdou Chekaraou M, Brichler S, Mansour W, Le Gal F, Garba A, Deny P, Gordien E. A novel hepatitis B virus (HBV) subgenotype D (D8) strain, resulting from recombination between genotypes D and E, is circulating in Niger along with HBV/E strains. J Gen Virol. 2010;91(Pt 6):1609–20. doi:10.1099/vir.0.018127-0.

79. Ghosh S, Banerjee P, Deny P, Mondal RK, Nandi M, Roychoudhury A, Das K, Banerjee S, Santra A, Zoulim F, Chowdhury A, Datta S. New HBV subgenotype D9, a novel D/C recombinant, identified

in patients with chronic HBeAg-negative infection in Eastern India. J Viral Hepat. 2013;20(3):209–18. doi:10.1111/j.1365-2893.2012.01655.x.

80. Michitaka K, Tanaka Y, Horiike N, Duong TN, Chen Y, Matsuura K, Hiasa Y, Mizokami M, Onji M. Tracing the history of hepatitis B virus genotype D in western Japan. J Med Virol. 2006;78(1):44–52. doi:10.1002/jmv.20502.

81. Drucker E, Alcabes PG, Marx PA. The injection century: massive unsterile injections and the emergence of human pathogens. Lancet. 2001;358(9297):1989–92. doi:10.1016/s0140-6736(01)06967-7.

82. Gerlich WH, Caspari G. Hepatitis viruses and the safety of blood donations. J Viral Hepat. 1999;6 Suppl 1:6–15.

83. Zehender G, De Maddalena C, Milazzo L, Piazza M, Galli M, Tanzi E, Bruno R. Hepatitis B virus genotype distribution in HIV-1 coinfected patients. Gastroenterology. 2003;125(5):1559–60. author reply 1660.

84. Pourkarim MR, Amini-Bavil-Olyaee S, Lemey P, Maes P, Van Ranst M. Are hepatitis B virus "subgenotypes" defined accurately? J Clin Virol. 2010;47(4):356–60. doi:10.1016/j.jcv.2010.01.015.

85. Coppola N, Masiello A, Tonziello G, Pisapia R, Pisaturo M, Sagnelli C, Messina V, Iodice V, Sagnelli E. Factors affecting the changes in molecular epidemiology of acute hepatitis B in a Southern Italian area. J Viral Hepat. 2010;17(7):493–500. doi:10.1111/j.1365-2893.2009.01201.x.

86. Wasley A, Samandari T, Bell BP. Incidence of hepatitis A in the United States in the era of vaccination. JAMA. 2005;294(2):194–201. doi:10.1001/jama.294.2.194.

87. Zehender G, Ebranati E, Gabanelli E, Shkjezi R, Lai A, Sorrentino C, Lo Presti A, Basho M, Bruno R, Tanzi E, Bino S, Ciccozzi M, Galli M. Spatial and temporal dynamics of hepatitis B virus D genotype in Europe and the Mediterranean Basin. PLoS One. 2012;7(5):e37198. doi:10.1371/journal.pone.0037198.

88. Mortimer PP. Arsphenamine jaundice and the recognition of instrument-borne virus infection. Genitourin Med. 1995;71(2):109–19.

89. Alavian SM, Fallahian F, Lankarani KB. The changing epidemiology of viral hepatitis B in Iran. J Gastrointestin Liver Dis. 2007;16(4):403–6.

90. Custer B, Sullivan SD, Hazlet TK, Iloeje U, Veenstra DL, Kowdley KV. Global epidemiology of hepatitis B virus. J Clin Gastroenterol. 2004;38(10 Suppl 3):S158–68.

91. Bowyer SM, van Staden L, Kew MC, Sim JG. A unique segment of the hepatitis B virus group A genotype identified in isolates from South Africa. J Gen Virol. 1997;78(Pt 7):1719–29.

92. Kramvis A, Weitzmann L, Owiredu WK, Kew MC. Analysis of the complete genome of subgroup A′ hepatitis B virus isolates from South Africa. J Gen Virol. 2002;83(Pt 4):835–9.

93. Sugauchi F, Kumada H, Acharya SA, Shrestha SM, Gamutan MT, Khan M, Gish RG, Tanaka Y, Kato T, Orito E, Ueda R, Miyakawa Y, Mizokami M. Epidemiological and sequence differences between two subtypes (Ae and Aa) of hepatitis B virus genotype A. J Gen Virol. 2004;85(Pt 4):811–20.

94. Kimbi GC, Kramvis A, Kew MC. Distinctive sequence characteristics of subgenotype A1 isolates of hepatitis B virus from South Africa. J Gen Virol. 2004;85(Pt 5):1211–20.

95. Hannoun C, Soderstrom A, Norkrans G, Lindh M. Phylogeny of African complete genomes reveals a West African genotype A subtype of hepatitis B virus and relatedness between Somali and Asian A1 sequences. J Gen Virol. 2005;86(Pt 8):2163–7. doi:10.1099/vir.0.80972-0.

96. Kurbanov F, Tanaka Y, Fujiwara K, Sugauchi F, Mbanya D, Zekeng L, Ndembi N, Ngansop C, Kaptue L, Miura T, Ido E, Hayami M, Ichimura H, Mizokami M. A new subtype (subgenotype) Ac (A3) of hepatitis B virus and recombination between genotypes A and E in Cameroon. J Gen Virol. 2005;86(Pt 7):2047–56. doi:10.1099/vir.0.80922-0.

97. Makuwa M, Souquiere S, Telfer P, Apetrei C, Vray M, Bedjabaga I, Mouinga-Ondeme A, Onanga R, Marx PA, Kazanji M, Roques P, Simon F. Identification of hepatitis B virus subgenotype A3 in rural Gabon. J Med Virol. 2006;78(9):1175–84. doi:10.1002/jmv.20678.

98. Olinger CM, Venard V, Njayou M, Oyefolu AO, Maiga I, Kemp AJ, Omilabu SA, le Faou A, Muller CP. Phylogenetic analysis of the precore/core gene of hepatitis B virus genotypes E and A in West Africa: new subtypes, mixed infections and recombinations. J Gen Virol. 2006;87(Pt 5):1163–73. doi:10.1099/vir.0.81614-0.

99. Hubschen JM, Mbah PO, Forbi JC, Otegbayo JA, Olinger CM, Charpentier E, Muller CP. Detection of a new subgenotype of hepatitis B virus genotype A in Cameroon but not in neighbouring Nigeria. Clin   Microbiol   Infect.   2011;17(1):88–94. doi:10.1111/j.1469-0691.2010.03205.x.

100. Pourkarim MR, Amini-Bavil-Olyaee S, Lemey P, Maes P, Van Ranst M. HBV subgenotype misclassification expands quasi-subgenotype A3. Clin Microbiol Infect. 2011;17(6):947–9. doi:10.1111/j.1469-0691.2010.03374.x.

101. Fujisaki S, Yokomaku Y, Shiino T, Koibuchi T, Hattori J, Ibe S, Iwatani Y, Iwamoto A, Shirasaka T, Hamaguchi M, Sugiura

W. Outbreak of infections by hepatitis B virus genotype A and transmission of genetic drug resistance in patients coinfected with HIV-1 in Japan. J Clin Microbiol. 2011;49(3):1017–24. doi:10.1128/jcm.02149-10.

102. van Houdt R, Bruisten SM, Geskus RB, Bakker M, Wolthers KC, Prins M, Coutinho RA. Ongoing transmission of a single hepatitis B virus strain among men having sex with men in Amsterdam. J Viral Hepat. 2010;17(2):108–14. doi:10.1111/j.1365-2893.2009.01158.x.

103. Hahne S, van Houdt R, Koedijk F, van Ballegooijen M, Cremer J, Bruisten S, Coutinho R, Boot H. Selective hepatitis B virus vaccination has reduced hepatitis B virus transmission in the Netherlands. PLoS One. 2013;8(7):e67866. doi:10.1371/journal.pone.0067866.

104. Kramvis A, Paraskevis D. Subgenotype A1 of HBV—tracing human migrations in and out of Africa. Antivir Ther. 2013;18(3 Pt B): 513–21. doi:10.3851/imp2657.

105. Andernach IE, Nolte C, Pape JW, Muller CP. Slave trade and hepatitis B virus genotypes and subgenotypes in Haiti and Africa. Emerg Infect Dis. 2009;15(8):1222–8. doi:10.3201/eid1508.081642.

106. Mulders MN, Venard V, Njayou M, Edorh AP, Bola Oyefolu AO, Kehinde MO, Muyembe Tamfum JJ, Nebie YK, Maiga I, Ammerlaan W, Fack F, Omilabu SA, Le Faou A, Muller CP. Low genetic diversity despite hyperendemicity of hepatitis B virus genotype E throughout West Africa. J Infect Dis. 2004;190(2):400–8. doi:10.1086/421502.

107. Andernach IE, Hubschen JM, Muller CP. Hepatitis B virus: the genotype E puzzle. Rev Med Virol. 2009;19(4):231–40. doi:10.1002/rmv.618.

108. Forbi JC, Vaughan G, Purdy MA, Campo DS, Xia GL, Ganova-Raeva LM, Ramachandran S, Thai H, Khudyakov YE. Epidemic history and evolutionary dynamics of hepatitis B virus infection in two remote communities in rural Nigeria. PLoS One. 2010;5(7):e11615. doi:10.1371/journal.pone.0011615.

109. Mello FC, Souto FJ, Nabuco LC, Villela-Nogueira CA, Coelho HS, Franz HC, Saraiva JC, Virgolino HA, Motta-Castro AR, Melo MM, Martins RM, Gomes SA. Hepatitis B virus genotypes circulating in Brazil: molecular characterization of genotype F isolates. BMC Microbiol. 2007;7:103. doi:10.1186/1471-2180-7-103.

110. Castilho Mda C, Oliveira CM, Gimaque JB, Leao JD, Braga WS. Epidemiology and molecular characterization of hepatitis B virus infection in isolated villages in the Western Brazilian Amazon. Am J Trop Med Hyg. 2012;87(4):768–74. doi:10.4269/ajtmh.2012.12-0083.

111. Alvarado-Mora MV, Pinho JR. Distribution of HBV genotypes in Latin America. Antivir Ther. 2013;18(3 Pt B):459–65. doi:10.3851/imp2599.

112. Venegas M, Alvarado-Mora MV, Villanueva RA, Rebello Pinho JR, Carrilho FJ, Locarnini S, Yuen L, Brahm J. Phylogenetic analysis of hepatitis B virus genotype F complete genome sequences from Chilean patients with chronic infection. J Med Virol. 2011;83(9): 1530–6. doi:10.1002/jmv.22129.

113. Torres C, Pineiro y Leone FG, Pezzano SC, Mbayed VA, Campos RH. New perspectives on the evolutionary history of hepatitis B virus genotype F. Mol Phylogenet Evol. 2011;59(1):114–22. doi:10.1016/j. ympev.2011.01.010.

114. Panduro A, Maldonado-Gonzalez M, Fierro NA, Roman S. Distribution of HBV genotypes F and H in Mexico and Central America. Antivir Ther. 2013;18(3 Pt B):475–84. doi:10.3851/imp2605.

115. Godoy BA, Alvarado-Mora MV, Gomes-Gouvea MS, Pinho JR, Fagundes Jr N. Origin of HBV and its arrival in the Americas—the importance of natural selection on time estimates. Antivir Ther. 2013;18(3 Pt B):505–12. doi:10.3851/imp2600.

116. Shi W, Zhang Z, Ling C, Zheng W, Zhu C, Carr MJ, Higgins DG. Hepatitis B virus subgenotyping: history, effects of recombination, misclassifications, and corrections. Infect Genet Evol. 2013;16:355–61. doi:10.1016/j.meegid.2013.03.021.

117. Kramvis A. Genotypes and genetic variability of hepatitis B virus. Intervirology. 2014;57(3–4):141–50. doi:10.1159/000360947.

118. Kato H, Orito E, Gish RG, Bzowej N, Newsom M, Sugauchi F, Suzuki S, Ueda R, Miyakawa Y, Mizokami M. Hepatitis B e antigen in sera from individuals infected with hepatitis B virus of genotype G. Hepatology. 2002;35(4):922–9. doi:10.1053/jhep.2002.32096.

119. Bottecchia M, Souto FJ, O KM, Amendola M, Brandao CE, Niel C, Gomes SA. Hepatitis B virus genotypes and resistance mutations in patients under long term lamivudine therapy: characterization of genotype G in Brazil. BMC Microbiol. 2008;8:11. doi:10.1186/1471-2180-8-11.

120. Kim BK, Revill PA, Ahn SH. HBV genotypes: relevance to natural history, pathogenesis and treatment of chronic hepatitis B. Antivir Ther. 2011;16(8):1169–86. doi:10.3851/imp1982.

121. Lin CL, Kao JH. The clinical implications of hepatitis B virus genotype: recent advances. J Gastroenterol Hepatol. 2011;26 Suppl 1:123–30. doi:10.1111/j.1440-1746.2010.06541.x.

122. Sanchez-Tapias JM, Costa J, Mas A, Bruguera M, Rodes J. Influence of hepatitis B virus genotype on the long-term outcome of chronic hepatitis B in western patients. Gastroenterology. 2002;123(6): 1848–56. doi:10.1053/gast.2002.37041.

123. Yang HI, Yeh SH, Chen PJ, Iloeje UH, Jen CL, Su J, Wang LY, Lu SN, You SL, Chen DS, Liaw YF, Chen CJ. Associations between hepatitis B virus genotype and mutants and the risk of hepatocellular carcinoma. J Natl Cancer Inst. 2008;100(16):1134–43. doi:10.1093/jnci/djn243.

124. Kew MC, Kramvis A, Yu MC, Arakawa K, Hodkinson J. Increased hepatocarcinogenic potential of hepatitis B virus genotype A in Bantu-speaking Sub-Saharan Africans. J Med Virol. 2005;75(4): 513–21. doi:10.1002/jmv.20311.

125. Warner N, Locarnini S. The antiviral drug selected hepatitis B virus rtA181T/sW172* mutant has a dominant negative secretion defect and alters the typical profile of viral rebound. Hepatology. 2008;48(1):88–98. doi:10.1002/hep.22295.

126. Araujo NM, Waizbort R, Kay A. Hepatitis B virus infection from an evolutionary point of view: how viral, host, and environmental factors shape genotypes and subgenotypes. Infect Genet Evol. 2011;11(6):1199–207. doi:10.1016/j.meegid.2011.04.017.

127. Livingston SE, Simonetti JP, McMahon BJ, Bulkow LR, Hurlburt KJ, Homan CE, Snowball MM, Cagle HH, Williams JL, Chulanov VP. Hepatitis B virus genotypes in Alaska Native people with hepatocellular carcinoma: preponderance of genotype F. J Infect Dis. 2007;195(1):5–11. doi:10.1086/509894.

128. Pezzano SC, Torres C, Fainboim HA, Bouzas MB, Schroder T, Giuliano SF, Paz S, Alvarez E, Campos RH, Mbayed VA. Hepatitis B virus in Buenos Aires, Argentina: genotypes, virological characteristics and clinical outcomes. Clin Microbiol Infect. 2011;17(2):223–31. doi:10.1111/j.1469-0691.2010.03283.x.

Chapter 3
Reproductive Assistance in HIV-Serodiscordant Couples Where the Man Is Positive

Rocío Rivera, Mª Carmen Galbis, and Nicolás Garrido Puchalt

Introduction

Human immunodeficiency virus (HIV) is a retrovirus that can be transmitted from one individual to another via unprotected intercourse (including anal and oral sex), via contaminated blood, and from an infected mother to her child (vertical transmission) during pregnancy, delivery or breastfeeding. This virus mainly affects T-lymphocytes, macrophages and central nervous system cells, as they exhibit the main viral receptor (CD4) on their plasma membrane [1].

R. Rivera, MSc • N.G. Puchalt, PhD, MSc (✉)
Andrology Laboratory, Instituto Universitario IVI Valencia,
St. Guadassuar Bajo 1, Valencia 46015, Spain
e-mail: rocio.rivera@ivi.es; nicolas.garrido@ivi.es

M.C. Galbis, PhD, MSc
Andrology Laboratory, Instituto Universitario IVI Valencia,
St. Guadassuar Bajo 1, Valencia 46015, Spain

Ophthalmology Investigation, Hospital Universitario Dr. Peset,
Av Gaspar Aguilar 90, Valencia 46017, Spain
e-mail: carmina.galbis@gmail.com

© Springer International Publishing Switzerland 2016   65
A. Borini, V. Savasi (eds.), *Assisted Reproductive
Technologies and Infectious Diseases*,
DOI 10.1007/978-3-319-30112-9_3

Acquired immunodeficiency syndrome (AIDS) is the most serious manifestation of a range of HIV infection-related disorders. The Center for Disease Control and Prevention (CDC) of the United States defined the disease in 1982, and since that time, a variety of definitions of AIDS, in addition to various classifications of HIV infection based on clinical evidence and laboratory confirmation, have been developed. Currently, the classification system is based on clinical, immunological and diagnostic HIV features [1].

It is estimated that there are over 33 million people infected and there have been 20 million deaths so far, with over 80 % of these infections transmitted sexually [2]. Many of these individuals are of childbearing age and the improvements developed in the treatments that increase life expectancy and quality originated in the evolution of protocols accompanied by the growth and expansion of assisted reproductive technologies (ARTs) that are employed to safely achieve successful parenthood in serodiscordant couples in which only one partner is infected, while keeping the partner and the offspring free of the virus.

The aim of this chapter is to analyse the currently available scientific evidence regarding the efficacy, effectiveness and safety of sperm-washing in HIV-positive men and its ulterior application in ARTs.

The Presence of HIV in the Ejaculate of Seropositive Males

From the beginning, HIV was characterised as a sexually transmitted disease, and semen from seropositive males has been identified as a transmission vector of HIV, although controversial results in early studies regarding the specific viral reservoirs within the ejaculate were published.

The presence of the virus in spermatogonia, spermatocytes and spermatids was demonstrated in pioneering studies [3]. However, this work was performed in atrophied testes from men who had died of HIV; thus, this situation is not comparable, and their conclusions not applicable to cases of men with low viral load and normal sperm count [4].

For decades, HIV has been identified as a virion (RNA) in the seminal plasma and as a provirus (DNA) in the cellular fraction of the ejaculate, knowing that HIV-positive men may have elevated levels of the retrovirus either in seminal plasma or in non-germ cells [4, 5].

The adequate characterisation of the viral reservoirs of the ejaculate is crucial, mainly in relation to the presence or absence of viral load in sperm cells, which are the specific cell types of interest to be employed to attempt conception. To this end, specific research on this topic has been conducted for years.

Although initially considered possible, as in the early 1990s several authors suggested that HIV might reside within the sperm cells [6–11] after the supposed identification of an HIV membrane receptor that was different from CD4 present in spermatozoa, resulting in doubts being raised about the possibility of safely using sperm from infected males for reproductive purposes.

The presence of HIV in the sperm was also detected in the semen of seronegative men after culturing in vitro with high concentrations of the virus [12], although in 1998, Kuji et al. [13], contrariwise, did not confirm the intracytoplasmic presence of the virus after the in vitro culture of spermatozoa with HIV.

Other authors have detected only the presence of HIV in the seminal plasma and/or in non-sperm cells in the semen (lymphocytes and macrophages), and occasionally in gametes, possibly because of an incomplete elimination of non-spermatogenic cells or seminal plasma, or an unspecific union with dead cells [14, 15]. They defend the complete absence of viral particles and nucleic acids in the sperm, showing that the separation of seminal fluid and non-sperm cells using the washing technique proposed in 1992 by Semprini reduces viral levels, as demonstrated historically by detecting viral particles using immunohistochemical techniques, but later increasing sensitivity by PCR and nested-PCR procedures, as discussed later (Table 3.1) [5, 15–18].

Table 3.1 Separation and human immunodeficiency virus (HIV) detection techniques in sperm samples from HIV-positive patients

Study	Sperm-washing	Swim-up	HIV semen detection
Semprini et al. [5]	Double-density gradient (40–80%)	Yes	Indirect immunofluorescence
Lasheeb et al. [18]	Double-density gradient (40–80%)	Yes	NASBA-nested PCR
Marina et al. [4, 19]	Triple-density gradient (50–70–90%)	Yes	PCR AMPLICOR
Chrystie et al. [26]	Double-density gradient (50–90%)	Yes	NASBA
Hanabusa [51]	Quadruple-density gradient (56–64–72–80%) in double tube	Yes	Nested PCR
Sauer and Chang [39]	Double-density gradient (47–90%)	Yes	None
Politch et al. [42]	Double-density gradient (47–90%) in a double tube	No	RT-PCR
Garrido et al. [34]	Triple-density gradient (45–70–90%)	Yes	Nested PCR
Mencaglia et al. [23]	Triple-density gradient (45–70–90%)	Yes	None
Bujan [50]	Triple-density gradient (50–70–90%)	Yes	HIV RNA PCR
Kato [52]	Double-density gradient	Yes	RT-nested PCR
Savasi et al. [31]	Double-density gradient (40–80%)	Yes	Real-time PCR
Molina et al. [45]	Double-density gradient (40–80%)	No	Real-time PCR

Factors Conditioning HIV Transmission Mediated by Sperm

Most infections result from genital exposure to semen of seropositive men, the risk of infection dependent on the number of virions and infected cells, the number and frequency of intimate contacts, the presence of other infections and genital lesions, the HIV infectivity, host immunological susceptibility and the type of sexual practice [19].

Furthermore, in relation to viral load, some studies suggest that blood plasma and seminal plasma might behave as different compartments, so that HIV can still be present and infective in semen even if blood levels remain undetectable [20]. This clearly points to the need to test sperm, instead of testing blood viral load, to assess reproductive options, and most importantly, to know that blood viral load is not useful in predicting the use for reproductive purposes of unwashed sperm cells.

Antiretroviral treatments may reduce blood and plasma virus levels, but RNA levels can still be detected in seminal plasma and non-sperm cells, supposedly because the diffusion and extent of antiretrovirals into genital compartments is quite variable, hypothetically because germ cells are protected by the blood–testis barrier, which prevents the entry of certain substances, including many drugs [21].

The risk of horizontal transmission in stable couples is considered to be relatively low, whereas it is higher when an individual participates in occasional encounters with different sexual partners. In comparison, the risk of vertical transmission from mother to fetus is in some circumstances is higher: a HIV-positive man can infect his child through the mother although there is no evidence of HIV transmission from a father through an uninfected mother to the child. The risk when both partners are HIV-positive is linked to the possibility of introducing a reinfection with different viral strains, which may worsen the disease status [22, 23].

In absence of safety measures in intercourse with HIV-positive males, virus transmission from man to woman is estimated to be roughly 1–3 per 1000 sexual acts [23–25].

Assisted Reproductive Technology
in HIV-Positive Males

At the beginning of the epidemic, the presence of virus in semen and vaginal fluids, the possibility of horizontal and vertical transmission, the high level of morbidity for prospective parents and children, and the risk of transmission to medical personnel led to the refusal of the reproduction specialists to carry out infertility treatments in this population [20].

With the introduction of highly active antiretroviral therapy (HAART), there was a delay and even a slowing down of the progression of AIDS, achieving extended survival and a better quality of life for people infected with HIV [1, 22, 24]. These advances have led the concept of the disease to be modified from being associated with short survival to the idea of the condition being chronic, with a similar life expectancy to other chronic pathological conditions, thus leading many seropositive people to have the possibility of becoming parents [23].

The HIV-seropositive males whose partners are seronegative may still have doubts about their paternity options, regardless of whether or not they are fertile, because of the risk of transmitting the virus to a woman through the semen via the unprotected intercourse that is necessary for successful conception, and also transmitting it to the conceived child [4, 26, 27].

Until recently, these couples were directed to sperm donation, adoption or abandoning their plans of having children [22]. The latter option is frequently not welcomed by these couples, mainly in countries where the other options are difficult or unavailable [28]. Improvements in the knowledge of the disease and in the field of assisted reproduction allow couples to form families under these circumstances and keep the risks to a minimum [20].

The immediate consequence of this situation is the need for an adequate reproductive counselling, enabling the options to achieve pregnancy in those couples where one or both partners are HIV-positive [29].

Although it remains a controversial issue, some authors still argue that under certain circumstances and with controlled diseases and infected patients exhibiting particularly clinical characteristics, natural methods should not be underestimated [30].

In addition, another important aspect to note is that not all of these couples may be fertile at the time they attempt natural conception, and one of the reasons for this may be age. Currently, males who suffered parenteral transmission due to drug addiction are usually in their 40s, and it is likely that their partners are also of a similar age [25].

In these cases, those opting for repeated unprotected sex in order to procreate may increase the risk of viral transmission, resulting in women becoming infected without having had a significant chance to get pregnant [27].

In this case, what needs to be carefully considered is the risk/benefit ratio, including the consequences of these acts in a scenario in which ART can avoid any hazard with almost 100 % safety.

The options that serodiscordant couples have for conceiving children when the man is HIV-positive and the woman is HIV-negative are related to undergoing sperm washing protocols, confirming viral absence in the washed sperm, and afterwards, using the appropriate ART with either artificial insemination or in vitro fertilisation (IVF) to reduce the risk of transmission using their own gametes from infected males [24, 29, 31].

Assisted reproductive technologies will allow the possibility of controlling the different stages of the reproductive process to minimise exposure to the virus and its transmission between the two members of the couple by avoiding intimate contact.

Semen Quality in Seropositive Men

Semen quality may be affected by HIV infection itself or the individual's overall health status [32–34], by the antiretroviral treatments employed [33, 34], and in the case of using ARTs to prevent horizontal transmission, by the process of sperm-washing, as will be explained later [1, 34].

Seminal characteristics of seropositive men have been the subject of many studies over the years. Several groups have compared semen samples from HIV-seropositive men with semen samples from healthy or HIV-uninfected men [32–34].

Some authors found changes in the pattern of sperm mobility, ejaculate volume and total sperm count [18, 32, 33]. However, in a paper published in 2005 by our group [34], no significant differences between groups were found, although a significant number of individuals (indicating enough statistical power) were available; thus, we were able to compare all the semen parameters between the groups, demonstrating that the variations found were not sufficiently marked to impair fertility, except for those extreme cases with a noticeable deterioration in health quality due to the illness.

The potential negative effect of antiretroviral treatments on sperm quality has also been the aim of several studies that compare sperm quality in men with different antiretroviral treatments (bi-, tri- or quadritherapies) and men with no treatment. These studies have shown that the use or not of antiretroviral therapy affects the sperm quality, the different parameters being comparable in the two groups [33, 34]. This gives an important message to family planners affected by HIV, in the sense that they will not need to abandon therapy to undergo ART because of a collateral fertility impairment.

Increasingly, there is information about the fact that the quality of the semen cannot be measured only by means of the sperm count and mobility assessment. In this regard, several sperm molecular factors have been related to male infertility [35, 36].

In addition, an indirect way of assessing semen quality is by evaluating the embryos obtained from its use, their quality and their ability to reach optimal blastocysts for later implantation and development. This methodology for assessing semen was carried out by Melo et al. [37] by comparing the morphological features of embryos from HIV-serodiscordant couples with infected males and embryos from couples with infertility associated with tubal factor mainly as controls, using intracytoplasmic injection (ICSI) for both groups. The results they obtained showed that fertilisation rates, cleavage and embryonic characteristics were similar in the two groups, finding no differences in the mean number of optimal embryos on day 3. When these embryos were cultured until day 5 or 6, a small but significant increase in embryonic arrest from embryos of serodiscordant couples was observed; however, the number of optimal blastocysts on day 6 was comparable in the two groups. Moreover, no differences in the number of cryopreserved and transferred embryos, implantation, pregnancies, multiple pregnancies or miscarriages rates between the groups were found. Thanks to these results, Melo et al. concluded that HIV infections in serodiscordant couples with infected males do not generate a significant negative impact on the developing embryo or in ICSI outcomes [37].

Regarding the relationship between HIV infection parameters and semen quality, the levels of CD4 and the viral count in blood are two of the most important values in describing the state of the disease. The decrease in CD4 blood levels is negatively associated with the duration of the disease [1], but did not seem to be related to sperm parameters. In this sense, low CD4 blood counts and a long evolutionary period of the disease are relevant factors for the sample, but are insignificant for the whole process of seminal-washing [34].

Many research groups found changes in sperm concentration in samples from infected men [18, 32], the total volume of ejaculate decreasing as the time since the disease was diagnosed increased, afterwards increasing the total concentration of sperm to the point of maintaining that number stable [33].

In 2005, our group [34] did not find changes in the sperm concentrations of samples from infected patients and also showed that as the disease evolved, sperm motility was not affected.

Sperm-Washing to Eliminate HIV from Semen

Sperm-washing is a sperm preparation technique, developed from the modification of classical sperm preparation methods, and has been available since 1992 in some assisted reproduction units to separate motile sperm from the remaining seminal components, following astringent methods to obtain spermatozoa without HIV DNA and RNA particles from infected males, aiming to eliminate or minimise the risk of transmission to the mother and baby when the sperm cells are employed in ART [5].

Before using, this washed semen needs to be analysed [38] to confirm the absence of virus in the treated sample by means of reliable molecular diagnostic tests, although some authors consider this confirmation step unnecessary because of the capacity of the procedure to diminish viral load in ejaculate [39].

In 2002, Sauer and Chang [39] published a paper in which they affirmed the increased security achieved through the use of ICSI in protocols of assisted reproduction in HIV-serodiscordant couples. In the methodology of their protocol they did not include the detection of HIV viral particles in semen samples after washing because they stated that the detection techniques used in laboratories showed low sensitivity. For this reason, they said that although detection is carried out before artificial insemination, the procedure was not without risk because a small number of viral particles could have remained undetected. This work has received several criticisms that claimed that although detection techniques were not extremely sensitive the solution did not lie in terminating its use [40]. Although the possibility of transmission is reduced through the use of ICSI, it is necessary to perform the safest method possible because the health of people is in our hands. In all cases testing for the detection of the virus in semen-washing samples should be carried out and those with positive results should never be used.

Semprini et al. [5] was the pioneer of the sperm-washing technique and published the first 29 cases of serodiscordant couples who had carried out ARTs after semen treatment by sperm washing. Fifteen women achieved term pregnancies without any seroconversion being found among them. This procedure provoked great interest and increased the hopes of many couples who wanted to have children without the risk of infecting the woman [5, 16, 17]. In fact, sperm-washing is the first method used to avoid HIV transmission in serodiscordant couples where the man is HIV-positive [29].

Such treatments today, thanks to all the studies and literature available, have been implemented in different assisted reproduction clinics and countries, yielding a high level of safety with regard to horizontal transmission and high success rates in achieving pregnancy [4].

This development is based on the demonstration that the viral reservoir within the reproductive tract and fluids are mainly located on seminal plasma and non-sperm cells, and therefore there is a huge reduction in the risk of transmission when using washed and selected sperm to inseminate oocytes [24].

Support for this technique is based on the hypothesis that the virus is not present in sperm, but is present in seminal plasma and non-sperm cells exhibiting CD4 receptors (classically for T lymphocytes and macrophages) [1].

Thanks to the use of sperm-washing and ARTs, a noticeably large number of births of offspring free from HIV fathered by infected males has been reported, which is the proof that this theory is correct.

Sperm-Washing Protocol

Although different variations of the sperm-washing techniques employed in different clinics exist, the elimination of HIV in raw sperm commonly consists of the application of a double and consecutive washing process for the semen sample, by means of slightly modified classical density gradients and swim-up [5].

These two techniques are commonly used in sperm preparation for human reproduction to isolate and select the most suitable motile sperm for fertilisation. The particularity of sperm-washing in HIV-positive patients is that the two techniques are used together and consecutively, with higher volumes employed in comparison with non-infected samples, an astringent protocol aimed at significantly reducing the risk of infection, compared with couples who try to conceive naturally [1]. Usually, only one routine sperm preparation is conducted in non-infected males.

The main variations in the sperm-washing technique observed between studies involve the different percentages of density gradients, time and centrifugal force, and the use of different methods to detect HIV after the sperm wash, although the spirit of the concept is the same: isolating only motile sperm.

Almost all authors report that they apply the technique initially proposed by Semprini in 1992, with small variations [5]. Some studies use discontinuous gradients with different concentrations [4, 14, 26, 41], whereas others use specifically designed double tube gradients [42], or do not perform the swim-up technique as a second step in sperm preparation [41]. Most of them, however, perform a combination of both methods: density gradients and swim-up (Table 3.1) [4, 14, 26].

Technically, taking the necessary precautions by keeping equipment and reagents in the specific laboratory to avoid accidental operator injuries with infected biological fluids may involve, among others:

- A vertical laminar flow hood
- A centrifuge with safety lids
- Incubators, pipettes, nitrogen tanks, microscope, etc. specifically designed for this kind of samples, avoiding cutting or sharp objects.

Specific recommendations will be provided in other chapters within this book.

An example of a specific sperm washing protocol may include:

• A first wash adding culture medium to raw semen in about 2:1 proportions, where the sperm is thoroughly mixed with medium, centrifuged (2200 rpm for 10 min) and the supernatant removed. The pellet is resuspended afterwards in fresh culture medium [14].

• Density gradient centrifugation: the technique consists of establishing liquid layers of different densities. To make a density gradient (Percoll®, PureSperm ®, SpermFilter®, Ficoll®) an isotonic solution is used, and generally (in standard washing), three layers of 50, 70 and 90 % concentration, made from a diluted version of the mother solution, are used to separate different sperm cell fractions. Then, the semen sample is added on top of the tube containing the preparation of gradients and is centrifuged (1700 rpm, for 20 min). Each component of the sperm begins to cross through the different gradients until it reaches the layer where the solution density is equal to its density, also taking into consideration sperm motility.

The speed by which each component is settled depends primarily on the cell size and shape, the smaller components needing more centrifugal force and more time to reach the same density layer than bigger ones. After centrifugation, motile sperm will be located in the higher density layer, that is, at the bottom of the tube. To recover motile sperm, the upper layers are removed to reach the 90 % concentration layer with the help of different pipettes or

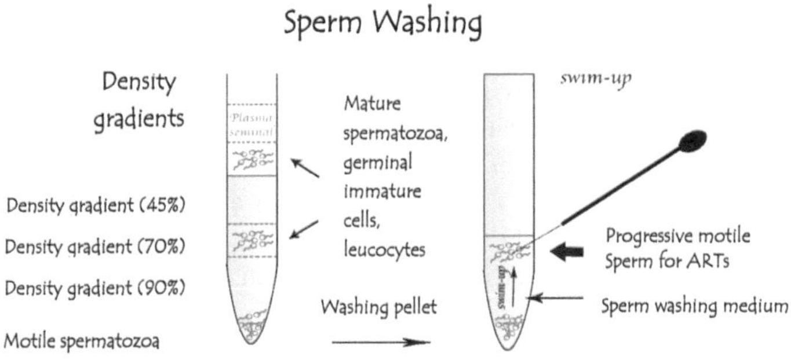

Sperm Washing

Fig. 3.1 Sperm-washing protocol

directly by reaching the bottom of the tube to remove the pellet below avoiding disturbance of the upper layers (Fig. 3.1).

- Swim-up technique: this is also based on the selection of motile spermatozoa. The pellet recovered after the density gradient centrifugation is placed in a sterile tube with a sperm preparation medium (e.g. Sperm Medium, COOK, Brisbane, QLD, Australia). Then the tube is placed at a 45° angle in the incubator with a temperature of 37 °C and 5 % CO_2 atmosphere for 1 h. After this period, the upper layer of the supernatant with motile sperm is carefully collected and transferred into a new tube, meaning that the result is about 1 mL of washed sperm suspension (Fig. 3.1).

The sperm sample obtained is divided into several aliquots. One of them (only 10 μL) is employed to assess sperm count and mobility, another to determine the presence/absence of HIV (one half of the total volume available after washing) with the different molecular biology techniques potentially employable, and the remaining (the second half) to be frozen by routine sperm freezing methods to use it later in the assisted reproductive treatment, after the confirmation of the absence of the virus in the washed sample.

The use of one half of the motile sperm retrieved with the seminal wash with nested PCR detection or other molecular biology techniques allows extrapolation of the results to the remaining fraction of the sample that will be later employed in ART, thus being almost 100 % sure of its safe use to prevent transmission, after the absence of a viral load in the analysed aliquot is confirmed.

The decision to perform double washes to ensure maximum virus removal adversely affects the amount of sperm available for insemination or IVF. It is necessary that these patients have an initially high semen quality, as after a double sperm preparation, only a low percentage of motile spermatozoa is found in the prepared sample, about 5 % of the total number available in the raw, unprocessed ejaculate [1, 34].

Nevertheless, special situations have been reported, and solutions raised in recent publications by our group, where the modification of the usual sperm-washing protocols, involving a less stringent method is described for samples with a very limited amount of motile sperm and even in testicular biopsy samples [5, 16, 17].

Undoubtedly, the theoretical risk of transmitting HIV with washed sperm should be lower than the risk observed in serodiscordant couples who have unprotected intercourse [27].

HIV Detection in Either Semen or Washed Sperm

The HIV belongs to the retrovirus family and has the ability to synthesise the reverse transcriptase enzyme, thus having the possibility of transforming RNA into DNA to be inserted into the genome within the host cell. In general, HIV detection techniques are based on the amplification of well-defined sequences of viral nucleic acids.

Historically, different techniques have been used to determine the presence or absence of the virus (Table 3.1). The first reports of women and newborns uninfected after the sperm-washing protocol and artificial insemination were published in Italy. Semprini et al. [5] performed HIV immunofluorescence detection for antigen p24.

There are several commercial methods for determining viral load, among them HIV RNA PCR (Amplicor HIV-1 Monitor; Roche Molecular Systems), branched chain DNA (bDNA; Quantiplex HIV RNA Assay; Chiron), nucleic acid sequence based amplification (NASBA; (NucliSense; Organon Teknika).

The first-generation techniques were only able to detect from 10,000 copies/mL. The most frequently used techniques (second-generation) have a lower detection limit from 200 to 400 copies/

mL [1], thus enhancing safety by reducing false-negatives. The detection method NASBA is a commercial method (third-generation) that includes a sequence as a control system to demonstrate the efficiency of amplification for each sample tested. Its sensitivity is as low as 50 copies per reaction [18]. Although this method has a low detection limit, the fact that a processed sample is negative, as with any analytical technique, still does not mean it is 100 % free of the viral load [26].

The most widely used method of detection is the standard PCR (polymerase chain reaction), consisting of the enzymatic amplification of specific sequences of the viral genetic material, allowing quantification of HIV DNA and HIV RNA from the motile sperm obtained by sperm-washing (proviral and viral load).

It is possible that standard PCR procedures may not be sufficient to determine viral levels in seminal plasma samples, because there is a limit to the number of copies that can be detected, and also because a specific protocol for nucleic acid extraction is necessary in semen samples, owing to the existence of polymerase inhibitors [25]. The sensitivity of the technique is usually around 200 copies/mL of RNA, estimated at about ten infected cells. It is possible that a few sperm contain HIV and it is not detected, but it is impossible to be 100 % sure, because the PCR is applied to a fraction of the sperm sample and the other fraction will be used for AI or IVF [4]. Moreover, in 2006, Persico et al. [43], compared in situ PCR vs nested PCR in unprocessed semen and in washed semen. They concluded that in situ PCR was inadequate for HIV detection, whereas nested PCR was recommended.

Currently, the technique that has proved to be more sensitive in determining the presence/absence of HIV nucleic acid in washed sperm is nested PCR. This method allows the detection of a single copy of viral RNA or DNA. With the application of this detection method, it has been shown that many samples that were considered negative using commercial detection methods were not completely free of viral particles [14, 40]. However, no reports of infection after checking viral presence using standard PCR or others have been published, and despite not being the most sensitive method that exists, given that very low levels, and thus few exposures are conducted, this difference between methods could be considered hypothetically harmless.

Prediction of the Result of Seminal Washing

Currently, there are insufficient data to show that certain sperm or disease parameters are able to predict the success or failure of seminal washing, to explain the small percentage of cases into which this procedure fails, forcing to the technique to be repeated to obtain sperm samples without the virus.

Positive results (meaning that some viral particles are still present in the washed sample) may be due to the inappropriate handling of the ejaculate during the washing process, leaving in the sample round cells or seminal fluid traces susceptible to carrying infective particles, such as lymphocytes and/or macrophages [27].

Nowadays, the only information that can be given to patients is the experiences of various research groups, and seems to point to the fact that the rate of positive washings may be around 1–5 % according to different reports. Moreover, the influence of the concentration and volumes of different density gradients used in the swim-up to give positive results is negligible [34].

Effectiveness of Washed Sperm in ART

Reproductive results obtained with washed sperm in assisted reproduction have been described to be comparable with those obtained in couples attending ART units for infertility and also exhibiting optimal embryo quality, depending on the age group, as expected for non-infertile couples [23, 25, 31, 37, 44].

Use of Artificial Insemination vs Intracytoplasmic Injection

Artificial insemination has been the initial method of choice for ARTs in HIV-discordant couples for decades when women's gynaecological tests and motile sperm count are compatible with a good likelihood of pregnancy [5, 19, 25, 45].

However, there are many cases, as with non-infected males, where artificial insemination use is not indicated, because of a predicted low probability of success in specific infertility cases, for example, in HIV-negative women with obstructed fallopian tubes, in men with low sperm quality or a low total number of spermatozoa after seminal washing, or even after repeated artificial insemination failure. In these cases, the use of classic IVF or ICSI is recommended [19, 44, 46]. Still, the use of ICSI is widely debated, apart from its classical use, as the systematic first choice to decrease the chance of infection when using sperm from seropositive males.

From a cost/benefit approach, although ICSI is more expensive than artificial insemination, the cost per child at home may be similar, and the total duration of treatment is lower [25]. The advantages of favouring ICSI rather than AI as a first option in HIV-serodiscordant patients are as follows:

1. The risk of infection with the use of a single sperm per oocyte is reduced compared with women who received millions of them in a cycle of artificial insemination [19, 20, 28, 39, 44].
2. Cycles are not cancelled if the sperm washed still has a positive viral load in a fresh sample (and the need to have a molecular biology result the same day). For ICSI, sperm remains frozen after washing, making it possible to repeat the HIV detection tests as many times as necessary until trustable results are confirmed, because the sample is processed before the cycle is started.
3. Pregnancy rates are higher in ICSI than in IA, as much as three times higher (generally speaking 40–45 % vs 10–13 % livebirth rates per attempt), reducing the time required for the conception and also reducing anxiety and stress for the couple facing this type of treatment and viral exposure with repeated cycles [20, 23, 39].
4. Optimising and making the sperm washing protocols and analysis profitable. The washed sperm, which is negative, given that has been frozen in small aliquots, can be used in different cycles, without the need for further washings, increasing the costs of the whole process.
5. It is not necessary to retrieve a large number of sperm to achieve appropriate pregnancy rates post-washing [20].

For these reasons, ICSI is the preferred and safest method used so far, because in discordant couples the possibilities of HIV transmission are reduced and pregnancy rates are maximised.

The obvious disadvantage of ICSI compared with insemination, when both techniques could be employed, are the side effects associated with these procedures in women, although some, such as ovarian hyperstimulation syndrome, seem to have been abolished in recent years.

Some authors have argued with regard to the possibility of entering unconsciously viral particles using the micromanipulation protocols, but to our knowledge, this point has never been demonstrated.

Although HIV infections have been reported when using unwashed sperm in IUI, [47], where 7 out of 199 women who were artificially inseminated with semen from HIV-infected donors (3.52 %) were finally seroconverted as HIV-seropositive. On the other hand, there is currently no information available indicating that washed and tested sperm can transmit the retrovirus, as clinical cases of assisted reproduction performed using a seminal wash, molecular confirmation of viral absence and ARTs, IVF, ICSI or IUI [31], no seroconversion occurred in neither mothers nor newborns, justifying the effort invested in each individual patient demonstrating the safety of the procedure.

Ethical and Social Issues

Sperm-washing followed by ART to minimise the risk of infection or horizontal transmission to the couple has generated some ethical and social dilemmas and concerns.

Given that HIV-infected patients have a chronic course of the disease and many of these patients are of reproductive age, to avoid infections, it is necessary to involve sperm-washing and some of the different ARTs that are available nowadays [1]. The ARTs in this case (serodiscordant couples who want to have a biological child) respond to the need to prevent infection rather than infertility problems.

There are in essence two concerns raised and reasons given for denying the ARTs in these couples: first, the risk that the child will be orphaned; and second, the possibility of the woman being infected and therefore the child. Regarding the first, the situation is exactly the same as with seropositive women: the survival period is extended because of the better control of opportunistic infections and the increased efficacy of antiretroviral therapy. The risk of virus transmission from infected men to seronegative women can be considered almost completely eliminated after sperm-washing and ARTs [22].

In 2001, an editorial entitled "HIV and infertility: time to treat" [48] provided arguments that led to debate and increased awareness of the problem. This editorial argued that there is no justification for denying treatment to parents who are HIV-positive: the use of antiretroviral therapy during pregnancy and childbirth, the caesarean delivery and avoidance of breastfeeding are proven measures that reduce the risk of vertical transmission to below 2 %.

In comparison, the risk of congenital malformations in newborns from HIV-negative mothers is 2.5 %, whereas this increases four-fold if the mother is diabetic insulin-dependent and ten-fold if she has a significant congenital malformation.

Currently, this disease is considered a chronic condition in which the life expectancy from the time of diagnosis in patients who receive treatment is over 20 years. Therefore, it is necessary to seek reproductive options for these patients. Nowadays, HIV-positive people are be able to have unaffected children and do not transmit the disease to their partners, although success is not guaranteed.

The authors conclude that couples in which one or both partners are infected should have access to the same advice and treatments as uninfected patients to allow them to conceive with a minimal risk of infection. Other alternatives can also be discussed, such as adoption, not having children, or sperm donation [20, 49].

Regarding HIV and health personnel, if the universal standard measures to prevent the transmission of infectious diseases are undertaken, the risk of HIV transmission is very small, and is not in itself sufficient reason to deny infected patients and their partners reproductive services [20, 26, 49].

Conclusions

To date, we can confirm, with the evidence available, that semen is a vehicle of transmission of HIV infection, although its presence in the sperm or germ cells, although a controversial issue that is still unresolved, seems difficult, given the low percentage of a positive viral presence after sperm-washes and the absence of infections in women and children. The sperm-washing, confirmation by means of sensitive molecular biology techniques and mainly ICSI are the most appropriate procedures for reducing the risk of HIV transmission in serodiscordant couples with an infected man, regardless of their fertility status, in a cost-effective and safe manner.

References

1. Oliva G, Pons JMV. Lavado de semen en parejas VIH serodiscordantes para su uso en técnicas de reproducción humana asistida. Barcelona: Agència d'Avaluació de Tecnologia i Recerca Mèdiques; 2004.
2. Halfon P, Giorgetti C, Khiri H, Penaranda G, Terriou P, Porcu-Buisson G, Chabert-Orsini V. Semen may harbor HIV despite effective HAART: another piece in the puzzle. PLoS One. 2010;5(5):e10569.
3. Nuovo GJ, Becker J, Simsir A, Margiotta M, Khalife G, Shevchuk M. HIV-1 nucleic acids localize to the spermatogonia and their progeny. A study by polymerase chain reaction in situ hybridization. Am J Pathol. 1994;144(6):1142–8.
4. Marina S, Marina F, Alcolea R, Exposito R, Huguet J, Nadal J, Verges A. Human immunodeficiency virus type 1—serodiscordant couples can bear healthy children after undergoing intrauterine insemination. Fertil Steril. 1998;70(1):35–9.
5. Semprini AE, Levi-Setti P, Bozzo M, Ravizza M, Taglioretti A, Sulpizio P, Albani E, Oneta M, Pardi G. Insemination of HIV-negative women with processed semen of HIV-positive partners. Lancet. 1992;340(8831):1317–9.
6. Baccetti B, Benedetto A, Burrini AG. Spermatozoa of patients with AIDS contain HIV particles. In: Melica F, editor. AIDS and human reproduction. New York: Karger; 1990. p. 47–54.

7. Baccetti B, Benedetto A, Burrini AG, Collodel G, Ceccarini EC, Crisa N, Di Caro A, Estenoz M, Garbuglia AR, Massacesi A. HIV-particles in spermatozoa of patients with AIDS and their transfer into the oocyte. J Cell Biol. 1994;127(4):903–14.

8. Baccetti B, Benedetto A, Burrini AG, Collodel G, Elia C, Piomboni P, Renieri T, Sensini C, Zaccarelli M. HIV particles detected in spermatozoa of patients with AIDS. J Submicrosc Cytol Pathol. 1991;23(2):339–45.

9. Baccetti B, Benedetto A, Collodel G, di Caro A, Garbuglia AR, Piomboni P. The debate on the presence of HIV-1 in human gametes. J Reprod Immunol. 1998;41(1–2):41–67.

10. Bagasra O, Freund M. In vivo and in vitro studies of HIV-1 and human sperm. In: Alexander NJ, Gebelnick HL, Spieler JM, editors. Heterosexual transmission of AIDS. New York: Wiley; 1990. p. 155–66.

11. Bagasra O, Farzadegan H, Seshamma T, Oakes JW, Saah A, Pomerantz RJ. Detection of HIV-1 proviral DNA in sperm from HIV-1-infected men. AIDS. 1994;8(12):1669–74.

12. Dussaix E, Guetard D, Dauguet C, D'Almeida M, Auer J, Ellrodt A, Montagnier L, Auroux M. Spermatozoa as potential carriers of HIV. Res Virol. 1993;144(6):487–95.

13. Kuji N, Tanaka H, Takahashi J, et al. Elimination efficiency of HIV from semen by Percoll continuous density gradient-swim-up. Hum Reprod. 1998;13:131. Abstract book.

14. Meseguer M, Garrido N, Gimeno C, Remohi J, Simon C, Pellicer A. Comparison of polymerase chain reaction-dependent methods for determining the presence of human immunodeficiency virus and hepatitis C virus in washed sperm. Fertil Steril. 2002;78(6):1199–202.

15. Quayle AJ, Xu C, Mayer KH, Anderson DJ. T lymphocytes and macrophages, but not motile spermatozoa, are a significant source of human immunodeficiency virus in semen. J Infect Dis. 1997;176(4):960–8.

16. Garrido N, Gil-Salom M, Martinez-Jabaloyas JM, Meseguer M. First report of the absence of viral load in testicular sperm samples obtained from men with hepatitis C and HIV after washing and their subsequent use. Fertil Steril. 2009;92(3):1012–5.

17. Garrido N, Remohi J, Pellicer A, Meseguer M. The effectiveness of modified sperm washes in severely oligoasthenozoospermic men infected with human immunodeficiency and hepatitis C viruses. Fertil Steril. 2006;86(5):1544–6.

18. Lasheeb AS, King J, Ball JK, Curran R, Barratt CL, Afnan M, Pillay D. Semen characteristics in HIV-1 positive men and the effect of semen washing. Genitourin Med. 1997;73(4):303–5.

19. Marina S, Marina F, Alcolea R, Nadal J, Exposito R, Huguet J. Pregnancy following intracytoplasmic sperm injection from an HIV-1-seropositive man. Hum Reprod. 1998;13(11):3247–9.

20. Ruibal M, Larcher JS. Riesgo de transmisión del HIV en parejas serodiscordantes en tratamiento de fertilidad. Reproduccion. 2009;24:115–27.

21. Williams CD, Finnerty JJ, Newberry YG, West RW, Thomas TS, Pinkerton JV. Reproduction in couples who are affected by human immunodeficiency virus: medical, ethical, and legal considerations. Am J Obstet Gynecol. 2003;189(2):333–41.

22. Englert Y, Van Vooren JP, Place I, Liesnard C, Laruelle C, Delbaere A. ART in HIV-infected couples: has the time come for a change of attitude? Hum Reprod. 2001;16(7):1309–15.

23. Mencaglia L, Falcone P, Lentini GM, Consigli S, Pisoni M, Lofiego V, Guidetti R, Piomboni P, De Leo V. ICSI for treatment of human immunodeficiency virus and hepatitis C virus-serodiscordant couples with infected male partner. Hum Reprod. 2005;20(8):2242–6.

24. Baker HW, Mijch A, Garland S, Crowe S, Dunne M, Edgar D, Clarke G, Foster P, Blood J. Use of assisted reproductive technology to reduce the risk of transmission of HIV in discordant couples wishing to have their own children where the male partner is seropositive with an undetectable viral load. J Med Ethics. 2003;29(6):315–20.

25. Garrido N, Meseguer M, Bellver J, Remohi J, Simon C, Pellicer A. Report of the results of a 2 year programme of sperm wash and ICSI treatment for human immunodeficiency virus and hepatitis C virus serodiscordant couples. Hum Reprod. 2004;19(11):2581–6.

26. Chrystie IL, Mullen JE, Braude PR, Rowell P, Williams E, Elkington N, de Ruiter A, Rice K, Kennedy J. Assisted conception in HIV discordant couples: evaluation of semen processing techniques in reducing HIV viral load. J Reprod Immunol. 1998;41(1–2):301–6.

27. Marina S, Marina F, Expósito R, et al. HIV y reproducción asistida. Reproducción Asistida en parejas serodiscordantes (hombre seropositivo) al VIH-1: experiencia de 118 niños nacidos sanos. Ginecología y Obstetricia Clínica. 2002;3(3):146–50.

28. Eke AC, Oragwu C. Sperm washing to prevent HIV transmission from HIV-infected men but allowing conception in sero-discordant couples. Cochrane Database Syst Rev. 2011;(1):CD008498.

29. Savasi V, Mandia L, Laoreti A, Cetin I. Reproductive assistance in HIV serodiscordant couples. Hum Reprod Update. 2013;19(2): 136–50.
30. Barreiro P, Castilla JA, Labarga P, Soriano V. Is natural conception a valid option for HIV-serodiscordant couples? Hum Reprod. 2007;22(9):2353–8.
31. Savasi V, Ferrazzi E, Lanzani C, Oneta M, Parrilla B, Persico T. Safety of sperm washing and ART outcome in 741 HIV-1-serodiscordant couples. Hum Reprod. 2007;22(3):772–7.
32. Dondero F, Rossi T, D'Offizi G, Mazzilli F, Rosso R, Sarandrea N, Pinter E, Aiuti F. Semen analysis in HIV seropositive men and in subjects at high risk for HIV infection. Hum Reprod. 1996;11(4):765–8.
33. Dulioust E, Du AL, Costagliola D, Guibert J, Kunstmann JM, Heard I, Juillard JC, Salmon D, Leruez-Ville M, Mandelbrot L, Rouzioux C, Sicard D, Zorn JR, Jouannet P, De Almeida M. Semen alterations in HIV-1 infected men. Hum Reprod. 2002;17(8):2112–8.
34. Garrido N, Meseguer M, Remohi J, Simon C, Pellicer A. Semen characteristics in human immunodeficiency virus (HIV)- and hepatitis C (HCV)-seropositive males: predictors of the success of viral removal after sperm washing. Hum Reprod. 2005;20(4):1028–34.
35. Garrido N, Remohi J, Martinez-Conejero JA, Garcia-Herrero S, Pellicer A, Meseguer M. Contribution of sperm molecular features to embryo quality and assisted reproduction success. Reprod Biomed Online. 2008;17(6):855–65.
36. Rivera R, Meseguer M, Garrido N. Increasing the success of assisted reproduction by defining sperm fertility markers and selecting sperm with the best molecular profile. Expert Rev Obstet Gynecol. 2012;7(4):346–62.
37. Melo MA, Meseguer M, Bellver J, Remohi J, Pellicer A, Garrido N. Human immunodeficiency type-1 virus (HIV-1) infection in serodiscordant couples (SDCs) does not have an impact on embryo quality or intracytoplasmic sperm injection (ICSI) outcome. Fertil Steril. 2008;89(1):141–50.
38. Garrido N, Meseguer M. Use of washed sperm for assisted reproduction in HIV-positive males without checking viral absence. A risky business? Hum Reprod. 2006;21(2):567–8. author reply 568.
39. Sauer MV, Chang PL. Establishing a clinical program for human immunodeficiency virus 1-seropositive men to father seronegative children by means of in vitro fertilization with intracytoplasmic sperm injection. Am J Obstet Gynecol. 2002;186(4):627–33.

40. Garrido N, Meseguer M, Bellver J. In vitro fertilization with intracy-toplasmic sperm injection for human immunodeficiency virus-1 sero-discordant couples. Am J Obstet Gynecol. 2002;187(4):1121. author reply 1121–2.

41. Dulioust E, Tachet A, De Almeida M, Finkielsztejn L, Rivalland S, Salmon D, Sicard D, Rouzioux C, Jouannet P. Detection of HIV-1 in seminal plasma and seminal cells of HIV-1 seropositive men. J Reprod Immunol. 1998;41(1–2):27–40.

42. Politch JA, Xu C, Tucker L, Anderson DJ. Separation of human immu-nodeficiency virus type 1 from motile sperm by the double tube gradi-ent method versus other methods. Fertil Steril. 2004;81(2):440–7.

43. Persico T, Savasi V, Ferrazzi E, Oneta M, Semprini AE, Simoni G. Detection of human immunodeficiency virus-1 RNA and DNA by extractive and in situ PCR in unprocessed semen and seminal fractions isolated by semen-washing procedure. Hum Reprod. 2006;21(6):1525–30.

44. Loutradis D, Drakakis P, Kallianidis K, Patsoula E, Bletsa R, Michalas S. Birth of two infants who were seronegative for human immunode-ficiency virus type 1 (HIV-1) after intracytoplasmic injection of sperm from HIV-1-seropositive men. Fertil Steril. 2001;75(1):210–2.

45. Molina I, Carmen Del Gonzalvo M, Clavero A, Angel Lopez-Ruz M, Mozas J, Pasquau J, Sampedro A, Martinez L, Castilla JA. Assisted reproductive technology and obstetric outcome in couples when the male partner has a chronic viral disease. Int J Fertil Steril. 2014;7(4):291–300.

46. van Leeuwen E, Repping S, Prins JM, Reiss P, van der Veen F. Assisted reproductive technologies to establish pregnancies in couples with an HIV-1-infected man. Neth J Med. 2009;67(8):322–7.

47. Araneta MR, Mascola L, Eller A, O'Neil L, Ginsberg MM, Bursaw M, Marik J, Friedman S, Sims CA, Rekart ML. HIV transmission through donor artificial insemination. JAMA. 1995;273(11):854–8.

48. Gilling-Smith C, Smith JR, Semprini AE. HIV and infertility: time to treat. There's no justification for denying treatment to parents who are HIV positive. BMJ. 2001;322(7286):566–7.

49. Ethics Committee of the American Society for Reproductive Medicine. Human immunodeficiency virus and infertility treatment. Fertil Steril. 2002;77(2):218–22.

50. Bujan L, Sergerie M, Kiffer N, Moinard N, Seguela N, Mercadier B, Rhone P, Pasquier C, Daudin M. Good efficiency of intrauterine insemination programme for serodiscordant couples with HIV-1 infected male partner: A retrospective comparative study. European

Journal of Obstetrics & Gynecology and Reproductive Biology. 2007; 135:76–82.

51. Hanabusa H, Kuji N, Kato S, Tagami H, Kaneko S, Tanaka H, Yoshimura Y. An evaluation of semen processing methods for eliminating HIV-1. AIDS. 2000 Jul 28;14(11):1611–6.

52. Kato S, Hanabusa H, Kaneko S, Takakuwa K, Suzuki M, Kuji N, Jinno M, Tanaka R, Kojima K, Iwashita M, Yoshimura Y, Tanaka K. Complete removal of HIV-1 RNA and proviral DNA from semen by the swim-up method: assisted reproduction technique using spermatozoa free from HIV-1. AIDS. 2006 Apr 24;20(7):967–73.

Chapter 4
Reproductive Assistance in HIV-Serodiscordant Couples Where the Woman Is Positive

Daniel Mataró, Rita Vassena, Oriol Coll, and Valérie Vernaeve

Introduction

The Virus

The human immunodeficiency virus (HIV) is an RNA virus discovered at the beginning of the 1980s [1] with a replicative cycle that can be divided into two phases: in the first phase the virus enters the cells [2], copies its RNA into a double-stranded DNA, and integrates this newly copied genome into the host cell. The second phase consists of the synthesis and processing of the viral genome, its mRNAs and proteins. Finally, the assembly and exit of the virus from the host cells occurs [3].

D. Mataró, MD, PhD • R. Vassena, DVM, PhD • O. Coll, MD, PhD
V. Vernaeve, MD, PhD (✉)
Clinica Eugin, Travessera de les Corts 322, Barcelona 08029, Spain
e-mail: dmataro@eugin.es; rvassena@eugin.es;
ocoll@eugin.es; vvernaeve@eugin.es

© Springer International Publishing Switzerland 2016   91
A. Borini, V. Savasi (eds.), *Assisted Reproductive*
Technologies and Infectious Diseases,
DOI 10.1007/978-3-319-30112-9_4

The most important characteristic of HIV is the destruction of the host's immune system [4], although neurological and tumorigenic properties are also often seen. The differences in clinical manifestations are due to HIV tropism of both macrophages and lymphocytes [5].

The high error rate of the enzyme reverse transcriptase, which plays a role in the process of retrotranscription of the viral genome in the host cell, causes genetic variability in HIV, and it is responsible, on the one hand, for a high proportion of defective virions, and, on the other, for the generation of a high diversity in the viral proteins, that allow for its escape from the control of a specific immune response [6].

Epidemiology of HIV/AIDS

Global data on the number of individuals infected indicate clearly the relevance of this disease. According to UNAIDS [7], 35.3 (32.2–38.8) million people are currently infected worldwide. In underdeveloped countries, the number of people infected by HIV is particularly high; in Africa alone there are around 25 million infected. This is because the chance of these people receiving adequate treatment is low there is a high level of infection transmission, sexually and vertically. This results in high HIV-related mortality. However, this problem is not exclusive to developing countries. For example, in areas such as North America and Eastern Europe there are 1.3 million and 860,000 people infected respectively, although their prognosis is better overall, because of the easier access to treatment in those countries.

Since the introduction of antiretroviral drugs, there has been a progressive decrease in the number of new infections worldwide, now 2.3 (1.9–2.7) million each year, a 33 % decrease since 2001, when the figure was 3.4 (3.1–3.7) million per year. At the same time, deaths have decreased over time, reaching the 1.6 (1.4–1.9) million mark in 2012, a marked decrease from 2.3 (2.1–2.6) million in 2005.

Women and HIV

Worldwide, a little more than half of the people living with HIV are women. Heterosexual transmission of HIV has been increasing steadily, and it is more frequent in women than in men [8].

Women between the ages of 15 and 24 are twice as likely to become infected with HIV [7]. The majority of infections are sexual [9] and most women who become infected with HIV do so because their partner engages in risky behaviour. In certain countries, a woman might think that she has no right to ask her partner to use a condom, even though she knows that he has had sexual relationships with other partners [10]. Research has repeatedly shown the relationship between sexual abuse and the risk of these women becoming infected with HIV [11].

If we look in detail at the transmission network, we see that, for instance, female sex workers are often intraparenteral drug users, and that a high proportion of their clients also have other sexual partners, whether spouses or stable partners; furthermore, many men who have sexual relationships with other men also have them with women, and the overall concept that emerges from this picture is that no mode of infection stands isolated from the others.

Fertility in HIV-Infected Women

Male fertility does not seem to be significantly affected by HIV, although it is hard to gather reliable data on the matter, as couples where the man is infected are recommended to have sexual relationships only with condoms and to try to achieve pregnancy using ART technology to minimise transmission. However, artificial insemination (AI) data from these couples indicate that the pregnancy rate is 26.2 %, whereas the pregnancy rate following in vitro fertilisation (IVF) is 37.2 % [12]; consequently, the reproductive outcomes of these serodiscordant couples are comparable with those of the general population.

In contrast, it is difficult to analyse the spontaneous fertility of HIV-infected women. Some authors report a diminished number of pregnancies [13–17]. An Australian study found that HIV-infected women had a birth rate that was half that of the general population [18]. One reason for this decrease might be the increased use of condoms in this population, with the objective of protecting themselves from infection, and also as a tool to avoid pregnancy. Another reason might be because of the lower level of sexual activity of women after receiving a diagnosis of HIV, more so if they are at an advanced stage of the disease [19]. Therefore, we could conclude that the decrease in reproductive outcomes in HIV-infected women is mainly due to changes in behaviour.

Following this line of reasoning, we may think that studying female fertility in underdeveloped countries might be less affected by women's behavioural changes, as usually there is less access to both contraception and pregnancy termination services. The diagnosis of HIV still affects women's behaviour [20], even though their desire to reproduce remains high [21].

A study carried out in Uganda, analysing the prevalence of conceptions, pregnancies and abortions, indicated a higher pregnancy rate in women not infected with HIV. Analysing women who were infected, but who had no apparent signs of disease, the pregnancy rate was higher than in those women with apparent signs of infection; moreover, the spontaneous abortion rate was higher in infected women than in non-infected ones [22]. A similar work carried out in Kisesa found a substantial reduction in natural fertility, even adjusted for age [16]. In conclusion, we can say that HIV-infected women do have reduced fertility, although it is still unclear whether this is due to changes in their sexual behaviour.

Therapeutic Management

Antiretroviral treatment, and especially the combined utilisation of these drugs, has caused a significant decrease in the incidence of AIDS and in the HIV-associated mortality, and has lowered the mother-to-child transmission rate; these events have created a radical change in the quality of life and life expectancy of infected patients. HIV infection has become a chronic infection and as a consequence both more and more infected men and women are considering the option of having children.

As HIV is a disease that mainly affects the population of reproductive age, and because the most significant route of infection is via heterosexual intercourse, the use of assisted reproduction technologies (ARTs) has become of central importance as a preventive tool. In couples where the woman is infected with HIV, the goal of ARTs is to allow for a pregnancy while at the same time avoiding transmission of the infection to either the partner or the child.

ARTs in HIV-Infected Women

In the context of ART and HIV, it is critical to know that all women who are infected with HIV, and who are therefore at risk of transmitting the disease while attempting to reproduce, are identified. For this reason, it is mandatory that measures are introduced to detect all infected women, which in turn will lower the risk of vertical transmission (between mother and child). Attention needs to be drawn to early diagnosis before conception and/or at the beginning of pregnancy; counselling needs to be available to women with the desire to reproduce, so that they can take action during the pregnancy to minimise the risk of their children being born HIV-free.

There are two distinct situations in this regard: on the one hand, we have citizens of countries with good access to antiretroviral drugs and good prenatal services. The good results obtained with antiretroviral treatments, the media coverage on infection routes and preventive strategies for vertical transmission have meant that increasingly, HIV-infected couples consider having children a real possibility. This is true in couples where both individuals are infected and in those where one of the members of the couple is infected. These are the cases in which we can apply all reproductive technologies developed to date to obtain pregnancies, while lowering the risk of vertical transmission (see below).

On the other hand, in developing countries, both the knowledge needed to avoid transmission and the access to antiretroviral treatments are low; therefore, it becomes of paramount importance to develop strategies focused on lowering the incidence of vertical transmission, regardless of the possibility of offering ART assistance.

Below, we detail the recommendations for medical professionals who attend to women wishing to reproduce, to pregnant women and to their newborns. These guidelines have been prepared and published by the expert group of the Secretaría del Plan Nacional sobre el Sida (SPNS), Grupo de Estudio de Sida (GeSIDA)/ Sociedad Española de Ginecología y Obstetricia (SEGO) and the Sociedad Española de Infectología Pediátrica (SEIP):

1. Evaluate the different options to obtain a pregnancy; among them ARTs, with the main goal of avoiding transmission, even if both partners are already infected by HIV.
2. If we encounter a pregnant HIV-infected woman, we need to know the most up-to-date protocols related to the use of antiretroviral drugs, both to improve the woman's health and to minimise as much as possible the risk of vertical transmission. This can be achieved with adequate management of both pregnancy and delivery.
3. Avoid an HIV-infected woman reaching delivery without being aware of her state of infection. To attain this objective, it is necessary to measure anti-HIV antibody in all women wishing to have a baby; if the woman is already pregnant, this analysis should be carried out in the first trimester, and regularly thereafter, especially in the third trimester, with the objective of identifying those who became infected while pregnant. If a woman reaches the time of delivery without knowing her state of infection, a rapid test should be urgently conducted to provide, if needed, the means of preventing vertical transmission during delivery of the child.
4. Develop an appropriate follow-up of the newborn, who will have been exposed to both the HIV virus and to antiretroviral drugs through the mother.

People infected with HIV resort to ARTs for two main reasons: an infertility problem or to avoid transmission of the virus.

Originally, HIV infection per se was considered to be a formal contraindication to reproduction, and ethically unacceptable.

Currently, this ethical debate no longer exists, and medical societies do not question the right of HIV-infected people to access ARTs [23, 24].

On the other hand, ART laboratories should update their set-ups to work with contaminated samples without the risk of infection for other patients. Health professionals should be trained to handle samples (oocytes, sperm and embryos), which must be handled under the assumption that they are contaminated. For this reason, everybody in the ART laboratory who is involved in these processes must have detailed knowledge of infectious diseases.

When evaluating which ART technique to suggest, the first distinction is based on knowing which of the couple is affected: the woman, the man, or both.

We also need to take into account the probability of HIV transmission when one of the members of the couple is infected, which in general terms is low [25], but which increases progressively with the viral load of the infected individual, or when there are lesions such as ulcers, inflammation, or abrasions in the genital area of the non-infected partner. This risk of sexual transmission is reduced while the infected individual is undergoing a combined antiretroviral treatment, and especially when the viral load is undetectable [26, 27].

ART Selection in the HIV-Infected Woman

Self-Insemination

An HIV-infected woman desiring a pregnancy does not need to resort to IVF as the first line of treatment. A simple way to avoid infecting an HIV man is to resort to self-insemination [24]. This procedure can be performed by the woman herself or by her partner, injecting into the vagina with a needleless syringe the sperm, which can be collected using a special condom without spermicide after a protected intercourse, in the fertile phase of the menstrual cycle.

Unprotected intercourse is not a suggested course of action, given the simplicity of the self-insemination technique. As discussed previously, HIV-infected women may be affected by subfertility; therefore, it is always suggested that a basic fertility study be performed, and IVF is recommended after 1 year of performing self-insemination that does not result in pregnancy.

Clinical Study of the Couple

It is important when evaluating the fertility of these couples not to delay their reproductive desire unnecessarily [28]. In the preparatory work-up for an ART technique in a couple where the woman is infected with HIV, we carry out the same explorations as if it were a non-infected couple, in addition to the following:

For both members:

- Cervical and/or urethral cultures (chlamydia, gonorrhoea)
- General analytics and serological evaluation (syphilis and hepatitis)

For the HIV-infected woman:
- Specific study of HIV, CD4 and the viral load
- Written opinion of the infectologist stating that the infection is controlled and that the risk of transmission is minimal for the non-infected partner
- HIV serology, which will be repeated regularly

Artificial Insemination or In Vitro Fertilisation

When deciding to perform an ART, the following aspects should be evaluated:

1. The stability of the HIV infection, together and in agreement with the infectologist, who is the reference physician for the patient. In the pre-conception consultation, it is important to explain the problems that might be associated with IVF, the risk of vertical HIV transmission and the possible drawbacks in the use of antiretroviral drugs during pregnancy.

2. The ART technique that is best suited for the situation, and the most adequate stimulation protocol taking into account the basic sterility study, the ovarian reserve, and the potential for the hormonal response of the HIV-infected woman.
3. The likely success rate must be discussed, and the fact that the results obtained might not be as good as hoped for [24].

Ovarian Stimulation

Before the beginning of controlled ovarian stimulation, a specific informed consent form must be signed to proceed with the ART technique, in which the general risks of the technique, in addition to the specific risk due to HIV infection, are described in detail.

There are no studies investigating which is the better stimulation protocol, or whether some stimulation drugs are better than others, or if we need to change the stimulation protocol in some way because of the HIV infection. However, all stimulation protocols in HIV-infected women need to take into account a likely ovarian resistance to stimulation, and that the need for higher doses of gonadotropins is related to lower pregnancy rates [29].

Ovum Pick-Up

The ovum pick-up technique is carried out in the same way as for any other patient, following the same protection rules to avoid infection of the personnel and of other patients.

Embryo Transfer

Some studies report that HIV-infected women present a higher rate of prematurity, growth retardation, preeclampsia and fetal death [30, 31]. We also know that there is an increase in the materno-fetal transmission when the membrane rupture is for longer than 4–6 h, especially if it is accompanied by a labour lasting more than 5 h [32]. Twin pregnancies are at a higher risk of prematurity [33]; therefore, ideally only one embryo should be transferred [34]. However, given the lower success of ARTs in these patients, it is suggested that a less restrictive approach should be used.

Oocyte donation cycles in HIV-infected patients provide results that are similar to those from non-infected recipients; oocyte donation can therefore be proposed and, in this case, the transfer of just one embryo should be carefully considered.

ART Outcomes in Couples with an HIV-Infected Female

There are some data available in the literature on ART outcomes in couples where the woman is infected with HIV. The first study of this kind was by Ohl et al. [35], in which the authors report a lower pregnancy rate in these couples after IVF compared with control groups, with a pregnancy rate per ET of 9.1%; subsequently, the same group reported a new study with a larger number of cases where the pregnancy rate was 23.9% [36]. In that same year, another research group reported ICSI results in HIV-infected women, with a pregnancy rate of 16.1% compared with 19.6% in control groups [37]. In 2006, Coll et al. studied couples where either one or both members were infected and who had undergone an ART [29]. After pairing by age with a non-infected group of couples, the authors compared women using their own oocytes for the ART technique with those who resorted to donor oocytes. This study allowed for a more comprehensive study of HIV and the effects of HIV treatment on reproduction. Six groups of patients were created:

Group I: Undergoing IVF, with an HIV-infected woman
Group II: Undergoing IVF, with an HIV-infected man
Group III: Undergoing IVF, where neither partner was infected.
Groups IV to VI: The same as for groups I–III, except that the couples were using donor oocytes for treatment

Results show that the couples in which the woman is HIV-infected (group I), had a lower pregnancy rate than the two control groups. Pregnancy rates were 16%, 45% and 40% for the three groups respectively. The numbers of biochemical abortions and spontaneous abortions were similar, as has already been reported in the literature [14]. The groups of patients receiving donor oocytes (groups IV–VI) did not show any statistically different pregnancy rates (40%, 56% and 49% respectively).

In 2006, Manigart et al. [38] studied 47 couples where the woman was infected with HIV and was undergoing ARTs. The pregnancy rate per artificial insemination was 25% and when the man was not infected, the pregnancy rate per transfer was higher than when both partners were (28.1% vs 12.5%). The study reported a pregnancy in two of the women receiving donor oocytes.

In 2006, Martinet et al. [39] published a study analysing the response to the stimulation of HIV-infected women and found that the pregnancy rates per transfer were 14%.

In 2009, Douglas et al. analysed 17 HIV-infected women, 14 of whom underwent IVF with implantation rates similar to their control groups (15% vs 19%) and three others achieved pregnancy through oocyte donation [40].

In 2010, Prisant et al. [41] analysed 52 couples in which the woman was infected with HIV and found no differences in the pregnancy rate per transfer compared with a control group in which the man was infected (17.6 vs 22.2).

In 2011, Santulli et al. [28] analysed 74 HIV-infected women who were undergoing IVF cycles. In 57 couples the man was not infected with HIV and they found clinical pregnancy rates that were not statistically different from the control groups (26.3% vs 36.3%). However, when the man was also HIV-infected, there were significant differences (12% vs 41%).

In 2013, Nurudeen et al. [42] reported an analysis of 36 HIV-infected women who were undergoing a cycle of IVF with partner sperm or donor sperm. The authors found no significant differences compared with their control groups in those cycles in women aged under 35 years ($n=8$); however, in women over 35 years ($n=52$) the rate of live births per embryo transfer was significantly lower among infected women compared with the control groups (6% vs 24% $p=0.04$). These authors performed 15 cycles in women receiving donor oocytes, with a pregnancy rate per transfer of 86%. It is relevant that in this study, 92% of women were undergoing antiretroviral treatment, their CD4 levels were very good, with an average of 707.1 Cell/mm^3, and all had undetectable viral loads at the time of the start of the cycle. The authors conclude that the presence of a well-controlled HIV infection does not worsen IVF outcomes.

Although the data available seem conflicting, it seems that HIV infection affects the results of ARTs; significantly, we do not know yet the mechanisms by which it occurs, nor do we know whether HIV affects reproduction by an action at the hypothalamic–pituitary–gonadal axis stage, the ovary, and the oocyte, or on the receptive capacity of the endometrium. The possible mechanisms for this are analysed below.

Possible Causes of a Decline in Fertility

While some studies discuss their results with oocyte recipients, only one work makes a comparison with a group with the same characteristics but without HIV infection [29]. This allows for the study of factors both before and after the embryo transfer. There were no differences among groups in terms of basal hormonal assessment, suggesting a normal ovarian reserve. However, women infected with HIV seemed to have an increased ovarian resistance to gonadotropins, which in turn may explain the decrease in pregnancy rates. HIV infection is not believed to affect ovarian aging [43].

Women infected with HIV respond to stimulation in a similar manner to the control groups, which suggests that there might be a similar ovarian reserve [39]. In the study by Nurudeen et al. [42] cancellation rates were 20 % owing to a low response rate and in Manigart's study [38], the rate was 42.9 %. Hence, the main source of low pregnancy rates might be thought to be found in the oocyte, possibly because of worse cytoplasmic maturation.

Mitochondrial Origin

It has been shown that nucleoside analogue antiretroviral treatments are toxic to mitochondria [44–48], and that the incidence of persistent mitochondrial abnormalities in the population exposed to antiretroviral therapy is higher than that observed in the general population [49].

Also, when follow-up has been carried out on children born to mothers infected with HIV who had treatment with antiretroviral nucleoside analogues, it was observed that there was a relationship between mitochondrial dysfunction and prophylaxis [50]. Likewise, a decrease in mitochondrial DNA and in their ability to become fertilised has been observed in the oocytes of women infected with HIV who underwent infertility treatments [51, 52]. These low levels of mitochondrial DNA have also been seen in the oocytes of patients with ovarian insufficiency [53].

As explained earlier, if antiretroviral treatments are able to affect the mitochondria, it is also reasonable to think that antiretroviral treatment might alter embryonic development and therefore the outcome of ART.

Viral Origin

Mitochondrial alterations as a cause of low ART efficiency are challenged when we analyse studies carried out in developing countries [17], where access to antiretroviral treatment is low and there is nonetheless a decrease in fertility. Moreover, women who received antiretroviral treatment succeeded in achieving pregnancy with greater ease [54]. Thus, we realise that it may not only be the antiretroviral treatments that affect fertility, but probably the infection itself, the HIV virus, the immune alterations caused by the infection or secondary diseases, that can alter the reproductive capacity of these women.

Therefore, it could be the virus itself that affects the oocyte. A study analysing the effect of time of infection, the highest viral loads detected during the monitoring of the infection, or the plasma viral load before carrying out the technique on ART results found no significant differences [29], nor has the presence of the HIV virus been detected in the follicular fluid of infected women undergoing an IVF cycle [55].

It has been long demonstrated that the direct penetration of HIV in mature human oocytes is not possible, owing to the absence of specific viral receptors on oocytes [56]. Although a report found that viral particles were present inside sperm and embryos by immunofluorescence, it is unclear whether HIV genes can integrate within the sperm genome, and whether the genes retain the ability to replicate in embryos [57].

Endocrinological Origin

It might be hypothesised that the impact of HIV infection on fertility might occur at the hypothalamic–pituitary–gonadal axis. Even after adjusting for age, BMI and drug abuse, some authors found no association between HIV infection and amenorrhoea [58], whereas others reported more alterations in menstrual cycles, oligomenorrhoea and amenorrhoea in HIV-infected women who did not have AIDS criteria [59–61].

However, analysis of the levels of FSH, inhibin B and the anti-Mullerian hormone in HIV-infected women found no influence on ovarian aging [43].

Immune Origin

Another work that analysed the association between the incidence of pregnancy and CD4 levels in the Côte d'Ivoire noted that the incidence of pregnancy was higher in women with CD4 lymphocyte cell counts above 350 cells/mL [62]. Finally, the study carried out by Coll et al. [29] concludes that it is the immune state of the woman at the time of undergoing ART that has more predictive power in terms of altered ovarian resistance and therefore, less chance of pregnancy.

After analysing the different mechanisms that can affect fertility in these patients we can say that before performing an ART, it seems important to have the infection as controlled as possible to obtain the best immune status, with good levels of CD4, and to do this, it is correct to use the appropriate antiretroviral treatment for as long as is required. We can therefore assume that the results of IVF in women infected with HIV can potentially be improved with proper treatment.

Pregnancy in the HIV-Infected Woman

Pregnancy in the HIV-infected woman has several specific aspects that should be known, both to ensure that her condition is properly managed, and to provide her with appropriate counselling when these couples face the decision about whether to get pregnant. Until now, the most important thing has been to prevent mother-to-child transmission and with antiretroviral therapy this risk has been decreasing, but other problems have appeared, such as its potential toxicity, obstetric complications, in addition to the limitations in the use of obstetric instrumentation or invasive tests.

Regarding vertical transmission from mother-to-child we know that the majority of HIV-infected children in the world have acquired the disease in this way. Transmission to the fetus may occur transplacentally during pregnancy, at the time of birth, or by breastfeeding through infected milk. If no preventive action is taken, the risk of transmission to the fetus is 14–45 % [63]. As the vast majority of intrauterine infections occur around birth [64], preventive actions can be undertaken once it is known that the woman is pregnant.

Factors Affecting the Risk of Mother-to-Child Transmission

1. *Plasma viral load*. This is regarded as the most important factor in vertical transmission [65–67].
2. *Maternal factors*. The clinical and immunological status of the mother plays an important role as those who are at advanced stages of the disease or who have low CD4 lymphocyte counts are at an increased risk of transmission [68].
3. *Fetal and neonatal factors*. Gestational age at the time of delivery is related to transmission, as prematurity has been shown to confer a greater risk of transmission [69].
4. *Obstetric factors*. All invasive procedures during pregnancy, such as funiculocentesis, amniocentesis, invasive monitoring etc., can increase the risk of infection to the fetus (British HIV Association guidelines for the management of HIV infection in pregnant women 2012. HIV Medicine). It has been shown that the longer the time between the premature rupture of membranes and delivery, the greater the risk of infection [32], although this does not appear to be the case when women have received antiretroviral treatment [70].

5. *Factors associated with breastfeeding.* HIV can be transmitted via breastfeeding; thus, there is a significantly increased risk of infection of the neonate [71].

In summary, mothers who do not follow any methods of preventing mother-to-child transmission, or who are not on antiretroviral therapy, but already present factors such as HIV infection at a symptomatic phase of the disease, low levels of immunity, high viral loads, preterm labour, invasive procedures, premature rupture of the membranes or who have a newborn with low birth weight, are all at an increased risk of transmission. Therefore, women with HIV should be informed about which interventions we should carry out to reduce the risk of transmission [72].

Interventions for the Prevention of Mother-to-Child Transmission

Identification of the Infected Women

The first step in prevention is the identification of the infected woman. The pregnancy control protocols should propose that all pregnant women, regardless of their risk factors, should undergo an assessment of the HIV serology at the first appointment with the consultant obstetrician (pregnancy monitoring protocol in Catalonia) [73]. If the result is not available at the time of delivery, a quick detection test should be performed so that, were it deemed necessary, it would be possible to implement preventive measures both at delivery and during lactation [74].

Use of Antiretroviral Drugs

The second preventive measure would be the use of antiretroviral treatments. In the ACTG 076 study [75], a decrease was observed in vertical transmission from 25.5 to 8.3 % with the systematic introduction of zidovudine during pregnancy, childbirth and with the newborn. Currently, the use of antiretroviral therapy has decreased the rate of vertical transmission to levels of around 1 % [76, 77].

Complications Using Antiretroviral Therapy

An important point to consider is the potential effects of these drugs on neonates. The monitoring of infants in the ACTG 076 protocol has not shown an increased number of congenital anomalies in the group of children exposed to zidovudine [78], nor have they shown a higher percentage of abnormalities in physical or cognitive development [79] or an increased occurrence of tumours [80].

Also, with regard to children exposed to antiretroviral treatment, a higher incidence of birth defects has not been observed in fetuses exposed either during the first quarter, or during subsequent stages of pregnancy [81]. Therefore, we consider that the benefits of the use of antiretroviral treatments aimed at preventing perinatal HIV infection clearly outweigh the potential risk posed by being exposed to them, as they diminish mother-to-child transmission, even with a low viral load; thus, the pregnant woman should always be treated [82].

Obstetric Procedures

Finally, it is advisable to minimise the exposure of the fetus to labour, reducing the number of hours between the premature rupture of the membranes and delivery, and to this end the practice of elective Caesarean section in untreated women would result in a significant decrease in the risk of mother-to-child transmission [83]. In deliveries in women with undetectable plasmatic viral levels and antiretroviral treatment, the risk can be considered very low [84]; thus, there has been an increase in the number of vaginal births [85].

Before performing an invasive technique or obstetric procedure, the risk–benefit ratio should be assessed, taking into consideration the environment and the resources available [29]; thus, the indications should be very restrictive [86].

In developed countries, formula-feeding should be recommended, except in those locations where this does not pose a greater risk to the child [87].

Pregnancy Outcomes in HIV-Positive Women

Women who have become pregnant and infected with HIV have practiced a greater number of voluntary terminations of pregnancy [18], but the number of women who decided to end their pregnancy has subsequently declined [14, 77, 88]. In relation to spontaneous abortions before the use of antiretroviral therapy, a greater frequency among women infected with HIV had been shown [22, 89].

Later, with the introduction of antiretroviral therapy, the results for these women presented specific rates of abortion, ectopic pregnancy and perinatal mortality equivalent to women who were uninfected [14], although a study from 1990 to 2006 shows a constant spontaneous abortion rate, despite the development in therapies [77].

However, it has been observed that these pregnancies have an increased incidence of preeclampsia and fetal loss in relation to the duration of treatment and infection [31, 90]. Also, puerperal infection [91] or thromboembolic complications [92] could be further increased in these patients. This necessitates stricter control in the management of these patients both during the pregnancy and postpartum.

Conclusions

The application of preventive measures and the introduction of antiretroviral therapy have reduced the incidence and mortality of this infection. Also, great efforts are being made to get these treatments to as many people as possible, especially in underdeveloped countries. However, even if a large reduction in the transmission of the disease were achieved, there would always be the risk of a resurgence of the epidemic until a fully effective vaccine were obtained [93]. Currently, mother-to-child transmission has declined significantly [94]; thus, the benefits of this desire to reproduce do not entail any problems with regard to the message of prevention. Therefore, it is medically correct to take action to make it easier for these couples to have children [95]. This involves adapting laboratories, trying to find appropriate procedures and useful protocols to achieve the highest possible percentage of children born without infection, and to make the message of prevention against sexual transmission more consistent. Therefore, when faced with a couple in which the woman is HIV-infected, the current status of the infection, the therapeutic possibilities, the risks of complications during pregnancy are all assessed and appropriate reproductive counselling is given.

The population of HIV-infected women has a lower fertility rate and when undergoing IVF a lower pregnancy rate than the uninfected general population undergoing IVF. On the other hand, if they receive donor oocytes, pregnancy rates seem to be unaffected.

In view of the suspicion that the immune status might play an important role in fertility, it is advisable to try to improve this status before the technique is performed, if necessary, using appropriate antiretroviral treatments.

References

1. Gallo RC, Montagnier L. Historical essay. Prospects for the future. Science. 2002;298(5599):1730–1. Epub 2002/12/03.
2. Freed EO, Martin MA. The role of human immunodeficiency virus type 1 envelope glycoproteins in virus infection. J Biol Chem. 1995;270(41):23883–6. Epub 1995/10/13.
3. Soriano V, González-LaHoz J. [Manual del SIDA. Vol. 6ª Edición]; 2005.
4. Perelson AS, Neumann AU, Markowitz M, Leonard JM, Ho DD. HIV-1 dynamics in vivo: virion clearance rate, infected cell life-span, and viral generation time. Science. 1996;271(5255):1582–6. Epub 1996/03/15.
5. Pantaleo G, Fauci AS. New concepts in the immunopathogenesis of HIV infection. Annu Rev Immunol. 1995;13:487–512. Epub 1995/01/01.
6. Pantaleo G, Demarest JF, Schacker T, Vaccarezza M, Cohen OJ, Daucher M, et al. The qualitative nature of the primary immune response to HIV infection is a prognosticator of disease progression independent of the initial level of plasma viremia. Proc Natl Acad Sci U S A. 1997;94(1):254–8. Epub 1997/01/07.
7. UNAIDS. www.unaids.org.

8. Marks G, Burris S, Peterman TA. Reducing sexual transmission of HIV from those who know they are infected: the need for personal and collective responsibility. AIDS. 1999;13(3):297–306. Epub 1999/04/13.

9. Global HIV/AIDS response—epidemic update and health sector progress towards universal access. Progress report. Geneva: World Health Organization, UNICEF and UNAIDS; 2011. p. 150.

10. Satande L. Sexual and reproductive health rights threatened through forced sterilisation of women living with HIV/AIDS: case studies from Namibia and South Africa. Toronto: Taking It Global; 2011. http://www.tigweb.org/images/resources/tool/docs/2649.doc.

11. Watts C, Ndlovu M, Njovana E, Keogh E. Women, violence and HIV/AIDS in Zimbabwe. SAfAIDS News. 1997;5(2):2–6. Epub 1997/06/01.

12. Oliva G, Pons JMV. [Rentat de semen en parelles HIV serodiscordants per al seu ús en tècniques de reproducció humana assistida. Barcelona: Agència d'Avaluació de Tecnologia i Recerca Mèdiques. CatSalut. Departament de Salut. Generalitat de Catalunya, Barcelona, September 2004]; 2004.

13. Willems N, Lemoine C, Liesnard C, Gervy C, Hien AD, Karama R, et al. [Is ovarian function impaired in HIV patients? A clinical pilot study in Burkina Faso]. Rev Med Brux. 2013;34(5):397–404. Epub 2013/12/07. La fonction ovarienne est-elle alteree chez les patientes seropositives pour le VIH? Une etude pilote au Burkina Faso.

14. Massad LS, Springer G, Jacobson L, Watts H, Anastos K, Korn A, et al. Pregnancy rates and predictors of conception, miscarriage and abortion in US women with HIV. AIDS. 2004;18(2):281–6. Epub 2004/04/13.

15. Ross A, Van der Paal L, Lubega R, Mayanja BN, Shafer LA, Whitworth J. HIV-1 disease progression and fertility: the incidence of recognized pregnancy and pregnancy outcome in Uganda. AIDS. 2004;18(5):799–804. Epub 2004/04/13.

16. Hunter SC, Isingo R, Boerma JT, Urassa M, Mwaluko GM, Zaba B. The association between HIV and fertility in a cohort study in rural Tanzania. J Biosoc Sci. 2003;35(2):189–99. Epub 2003/04/01.

17. Lewis JJ, Ronsmans C, Ezeh A, Gregson S. The population impact of HIV on fertility in sub-Saharan Africa. AIDS. 2004;18 Suppl 2:S35–43. Epub 2004/08/21.

18. Thackway SV, Furner V, Mijch A, Cooper DA, Holland D, Martinez P, et al. Fertility and reproductive choice in women with HIV-1 infection. AIDS. 1997;11(5):663–7. Epub 1997/04/01.

19. Roche N, Kahn M, Mathur-Wagh U, Wilets I, King K, Stein JH. Sexual activity in a cohort of HIV-1 positive women. HIV infection in

women: setting a new agenda conference, Washington, DC, February 1995 [Abstract WP-360]; 1995.

20. Wekesa E, Coast E. Living with HIV postdiagnosis: a qualitative study of the experiences of Nairobi slum residents. BMJ Open. 2013;3(5). Epub 2013/05/07.

21. Mmbaga EJ, Leyna GH, Ezekiel MJ, Kakoko DC. Fertility desire and intention of people living with HIV/AIDS in Tanzania: a call for restructuring care and treatment services. BMC Public Health. 2013;13:86. Epub 2013/01/31.

22. Gray RH, Wawer MJ, Serwadda D, Sewankambo N, Li C, Wabwire-Mangen F, et al. Population-based study of fertility in women with HIV-1 infection in Uganda. Lancet. 1998;351(9096):98–103. Epub 1998/01/24.

23. Human immunodeficiency virus (HIV) and infertility treatment: a committee opinion. Ethics Committee of the American Society for Reproductive Medicine; Fertility and Sterility 2015 Jul; 104(1):e1-8. doi:10.1016/j.fertnstert.2015.04.004.

24. Gout C, Rougier N, Oger P, Dorphin B, Kahn V, Jacquesson L, et al. [Assisted Reproductive Technologies in HIV patients: a comprehensive review of indications, techniques and results]. Gynecol Obstet Fertil. 2011;39(12):704–8. Epub 2011/08/30. Assistance medicale a la procreation et VIH: revue des indications, techniques et resultats.

25. Mandelbrot L, Heard I, Henrion-Geant E, Henrion R. Natural conception in HIV-negative women with HIV-infected partners. Lancet. 1997;349(9055):850–1. Epub 1997/03/22.

26. Wilson DP, Law MG, Grulich AE, Cooper DA, Kaldor JM. Relation between HIV viral load and infectiousness: a model-based analysis. Lancet. 2008;372(9635):314–20. Epub 2008/07/29.

27. Cohen MS, Chen YQ, McCauley M, Gamble T, Hosseinipour MC, Kumarasamy N, et al. Prevention of HIV-1 infection with early antiretroviral therapy. N Engl J Med. 2011;365(6):493–505. Epub 2011/07/20.

28. Santulli P, Gayet V, Fauque P, Chopin N, Dulioust E, Wolf JP, et al. HIV-positive patients undertaking ART have longer infertility histories than age-matched control subjects. Fertil Steril. 2011;95(2):507–12. Epub 2010/10/26.

29. Coll O, Suy A, Figueras F, Vernaeve V, Martinez E, Mataro D, et al. Decreased pregnancy rate after in-vitro fertilization in HIV-infected women receiving HAART. AIDS. 2006;20(1):121–3. Epub 2005/12/06.

30. European Collaborative Study, Swiss Mother and Child HIV Cohort Study. Combination antiretroviral therapy and duration of pregnancy. AIDS. 2000;14(18):2913–20. Epub 2001/06/12.

31. Suy A, Martinez E, Coll O, Lonca M, Palacio M, de Lazzari E, et al. Increased risk of pre-eclampsia and fetal death in HIV-infected pregnant women receiving highly active antiretroviral therapy. AIDS. 2006;20(1):59–66. Epub 2005/12/06.

32. Garcia-Tejedor A, Perales A, Maiques V. Duration of ruptured membranes and extended labor are risk factors for HIV transmission. Int J Gynaecol Obstet. 2003;82(1):17–23. Epub 2003/07/02.

33. Rode L, Tabor A. Prevention of preterm delivery in twin pregnancy. Best Pract Res Clin Obstet Gynaecol. 2014;28(2):273–83. Epub 2014/01/01.

34. Sunderam S, Kissin DM, Crawford S, Anderson JE, Folger SG, Jamieson DJ, et al. Assisted reproductive technology surveillance – United States, 2010. Morb Mortal Wkly Rep Surveill Summ. 2013;62(9):1–24. Epub 2013/12/12.

35. Ohl J, Partisani M, Wittemer C, Schmitt MP, Cranz C, Stoll-Keller F, et al. Assisted reproduction techniques for HIV serodiscordant couples: 18 months of experience. Hum Reprod. 2003;18(6):1244–9. Epub 2003/05/30.

36. Ohl J, Partisani M, Wittemer C, Lang JM, Viville S, Favre R. Encouraging results despite complexity of multidisciplinary care of HIV-infected women using assisted reproduction techniques. Hum Reprod. 2005;20(11):3136–40. Epub 2005/07/12.

37. Terriou P, Auquier P, Chabert-Orsini V, Chinchole JM, Cravello L, Giorgetti C, et al. Outcome of ICSI in HIV-1-infected women. Hum Reprod. 2005;20(10):2838–43. Epub 2005/06/28.

38. Manigart Y, Rozenberg S, Barlow P, Gerard M, Bertrand E, Delvigne A. ART outcome in HIV-infected patients. Hum Reprod. 2006;21(11):2935–40. Epub 2006/08/05.

39. Martinet V, Manigart Y, Rozenberg S, Becker B, Gerard M, Delvigne A. Ovarian response to stimulation of HIV-positive patients during IVF treatment: a matched, controlled study. Hum Reprod. 2006;21(5):1212–7. Epub 2006/01/28.

40. Douglas NC, Wang JG, Yu B, Gaddipati S, Guarnaccia MM, Sauer MV. A systematic, multidisciplinary approach to address the reproductive needs of HIV-seropositive women. Reprod Biomed Online. 2009;19(2):257–63. Epub 2009/08/29.

41. Prisant N, Tubiana R, Lefebvre G, Lebray P, Marcelin AG, Thibault V, et al. HIV-1 or hepatitis C chronic infection in serodiscordant infertile couples has no impact on infertility treatment outcome. Fertil Steril. 2010;93(3):1020–3. Epub 2009/09/08.

42. Nurudeen SK, Grossman LC, Bourne L, Guarnaccia MM, Sauer MV, Douglas NC. Reproductive outcomes of HIV seropositive women

treated by assisted reproduction. J Womens Health. 2013;22(3):243–9. Epub 2013/02/27.

43. Seifer DB, Golub ET, Lambert-Messerlian G, Springer G, Holman S, Moxley M, et al. Biologic markers of ovarian reserve and reproductive aging: application in a cohort study of HIV infection in women. Fertil Steril. 2007;88(6):1645–52. Epub 2007/04/10.

44. Dalakas MC, Illa I, Pezeshkpour GH, Laukaitis JP, Cohen B, Griffin JL. Mitochondrial myopathy caused by long-term zidovudine therapy. N Engl J Med. 1990;322(16):1098–105. Epub 1990/04/19.

45. Arnaudo E, Dalakas M, Shanske S, Moraes CT, DiMauro S, Schon EA. Depletion of muscle mitochondrial DNA in AIDS patients with zidovudine-induced myopathy. Lancet. 1991;337(8740):508–10. Epub 1991/03/02.

46. Brinkman K, Kakuda TN. Mitochondrial toxicity of nucleoside analogue reverse transcriptase inhibitors: a looming obstacle for long-term antiretroviral therapy? Curr Opin Infect Dis. 2000;13(1):5–11. Epub 2002/04/20.

47. Kohler JJ, Lewis W. A brief overview of mechanisms of mitochondrial toxicity from NRTIs. Environ Mol Mutagen. 2007;48(3–4):166–72. Epub 2006/06/08.

48. Lewis W, Dalakas MC. Mitochondrial toxicity of antiviral drugs. Nat Med. 1995;1(5):417–22. Epub 1995/05/01.

49. Barret B, Tardieu M, Rustin P, Lacroix C, Chabrol B, Desguerre I, et al. Persistent mitochondrial dysfunction in HIV-1-exposed but uninfected infants: clinical screening in a large prospective cohort. AIDS. 2003;17(12):1769–85. Epub 2003/08/02.

50. Blanche S, Tardieu M, Rustin P, Slama A, Barret B, Firtion G, et al. Persistent mitochondrial dysfunction and perinatal exposure to antiretroviral nucleoside analogues. Lancet. 1999;354(9184):1084–9. Epub 1999/10/06.

51. Lopez S, Coll O, Durban M, Hernandez S, Vidal R, Suy A, et al. Mitochondrial DNA depletion in oocytes of HIV-infected antiretroviral-treated infertile women. Antivir Ther. 2008;13(6):833–8. Epub 2008/10/09.

52. Reynier P, May-Panloup P, Chretien MF, Morgan CJ, Jean M, Savagner F, et al. Mitochondrial DNA content affects the fertilizability of human oocytes. Mol Hum Reprod. 2001;7(5):425–9. Epub 2001/05/02.

53. May-Panloup P, Chretien MF, Jacques C, Vasseur C, Malthiery Y, Reynier P. Low oocyte mitochondrial DNA content in ovarian insufficiency. Hum Reprod. 2005;20(3):593–7. Epub 2004/12/21.

54. Myer L, Carter RJ, Katyal M, Toro P, El-Sadr WM, Abrams EJ. Impact of antiretroviral therapy on incidence of pregnancy among HIV-infected women in Sub-Saharan Africa: a cohort study. PLoS Med. 2010;7(2):e1000229. Epub 2010/02/18.

55. Bertrand E, Zissis G, Marissens D, Gerard M, Rozenberg S, Barlow P, et al. Presence of HIV-1 in follicular fluids, flushes and cumulus oophorus cells of HIV-1-seropositive women during assisted-reproduction technology. AIDS. 2004;18(5):823–5. Epub 2004/04/13.

56. Baccetti B, Benedetto A, Collodel G, di Caro A, Garbuglia AR, Piomboni P. The debate on the presence of HIV-1 in human gametes. J Reprod Immunol. 1998;41(1–2):41–67. Epub 1999/04/23.

57. Wang D, Li LB, Hou ZW, Kang XJ, Xie QD, Yu XJ, et al. The integrated HIV-1 provirus in patient sperm chromosome and its transfer into the early embryo by fertilization. PLoS One. 2011;6(12):e28586. Epub 2011/12/24.

58. Ellerbrok H, Fleischer C, Vandamme AM, Kucherer C, Pauli G. Sequence analysis of two HTLV type I infections imported to Germany. AIDS Res Hum Retroviruses. 1997;13(14):1255–8. Epub 1997/10/06.

59. Lo JC, Schambelan M. Reproductive function in human immunodeficiency virus infection. J Clin Endocrinol Metab. 2001;86(6):2338–43. Epub 2001/06/09.

60. Chirgwin KD, Feldman J, Muneyyirci-Delale O, Landesman S, Minkoff H. Menstrual function in human immunodeficiency virus-infected women without acquired immunodeficiency syndrome. J Acquir Immune Defic Syndr Hum Retrovirol. 1996;12(5):489–94. Epub 1996/08/15.

61. Cejtin HE, Kalinowski A, Bacchetti P, Taylor RN, Watts DH, Kim S, et al. Effects of human immunodeficiency virus on protracted amenorrhea and ovarian dysfunction. Obstet Gynecol. 2006;108(6):1423–31. Epub 2006/12/02.

62. Loko MA, Toure S, Dakoury-Dogbo N, Gabillard D, Leroy V, Anglaret X. Decreasing incidence of pregnancy by decreasing CD4 cell count in HIV-infected women in Cote d'Ivoire: a 7-year cohort study. AIDS. 2005;19(4):443–5. Epub 2005/03/08.

63. Coll O, Fiore S, Floridia M, Giaquinto C, Grosch-Worner I, Guiliano M, et al. Pregnancy and HIV infection: a European consensus on management. AIDS. 2002;16 Suppl 2:S1–18. Epub 2002/12/14.

64. McGowan JP, Shah SS. Prevention of perinatal HIV transmission during pregnancy. J Antimicrob Chemother. 2000;46(5):657–68. Epub 2000/11/04.

65. Coll O, Hernandez M, Boucher CA, Fortuny C, de Tejada BM, Canet Y, et al. Vertical HIV-1 transmission correlates with a high maternal viral load at delivery. J Acquir Immune Defic Syndr Hum Retrovirol. 1997;14(1):26–30. Epub 1997/01/01.

66. Mofenson LM, Harris DR, Rich K, Meyer 3rd WA, Read JS, Moye Jr J, et al. Serum HIV-1 p24 antibody, HIV-1 RNA copy number and CD4 lymphocyte percentage are independently associated with risk of mortality in HIV-1-infected children. National Institute of Child Health and Human Development Intravenous Immunoglobulin Clinical Trial Study Group. AIDS. 1999;13(1):31–9. Epub 1999/04/20.

67. Garcia PM, Kalish LA, Pitt J, Minkoff H, Quinn TC, Burchett SK, et al. Maternal levels of plasma human immunodeficiency virus type 1 RNA and the risk of perinatal transmission. Women and Infants Transmission Study Group. N Engl J Med. 1999;341(6):394–402. Epub 1999/08/05.

68. Fawzi W, Msamanga G, Renjifo B, Spiegelman D, Urassa E, Hashemi L, et al. Predictors of intrauterine and intrapartum transmission of HIV-1 among Tanzanian women. AIDS. 2001;15(9):1157–65. Epub 2001/06/21.

69. European Collaborative Study, Boer K, England K, Godfried MH, Thorne C. Mode of delivery in HIV-infected pregnant women and prevention of mother-to-child transmission: changing practices in Western Europe. HIV Med. 2010;11(6):368–78. Epub 2010/01/12.

70. Cotter AM, Brookfield KF, Duthely LM, Gonzalez Quintero VH, Potter JE, O'Sullivan MJ. Duration of membrane rupture and risk of perinatal transmission of HIV-1 in the era of combination antiretroviral therapy. Am J Obstet Gynecol. 2012;207(6):482.e1–5. Epub 2012/10/30.

71. Breastfeeding and HIV International Transmission Study Group, Coutsoudis A, Dabis F, Fawzi W, Gaillard P, et al. Late postnatal transmission of HIV-1 in breast-fed children: an individual patient data meta-analysis. J Infect Dis. 2004;189(12):2154–66. Epub 2004/06/08.

72. Grupo de expertos de la Secretaría del Plan Nacional sobre el Sida (SPNS) GdEdSGSEdGyOSyS. [Guía práctica para el seguimiento de la infección por VIH en relación con la reproducción, embarazo, parto y profilaxis de la transmisión vertical del niño expuesto]; 2013.

73. Iribarren JA, Ramos JT, Guerra L, Coll O, de Jose MI, Domingo P, et al. [Prevention of vertical transmission and treatment of infection caused by the human immunodeficiency virus in the pregnant woman. Recommendations of the Study Group for AIDS, Infectious Diseases, and Clinical Microbiology, the Spanish Pediatric Association, the National AIDS Plan and the Spanish Gynecology and Obstetrics

Society]. Enferm Infecc Microbiol Clin. 2001;19(7):314–35. Epub 2001/12/19. Prevencion de la transmision vertical y tratamiento de la infeccion por el virus de la inmunodeficiencia humana en la mujer embarazada. Recommendaciones de GESIDA-SEIMC, AEP, PNS, y SEGO.

74. Bulterys M, Fowler MG, Van Rompay KK, Kourtis AP. Prevention of mother-to-child transmission of HIV-1 through breast-feeding: past, present, and future. J Infect Dis. 2004;189(12):2149–53. Epub 2004/06/08.

75. Connor EM, Sperling RS, Gelber R, Kiselev P, Scott G, O'Sullivan MJ, et al. Reduction of maternal-infant transmission of human immunodeficiency virus type 1 with zidovudine treatment. Pediatric AIDS Clinical Trials Group Protocol 076 Study Group. N Engl J Med. 1994;331(18):1173–80. Epub 1994/11/03.

76. European Collaborative Study. Mother-to-child transmission of HIV infection in the era of highly active antiretroviral therapy. Clin Infect Dis. 2005;40(3):458–65. Epub 2005/01/26.

77. Townsend CL, Cortina-Borja M, Peckham CS, de Ruiter A, Lyall H, Tookey PA. Low rates of mother-to-child transmission of HIV following effective pregnancy interventions in the United Kingdom and Ireland, 2000-2006. AIDS. 2008;22(8):973–81. Epub 2008/05/06.

78. Sperling RS, Shapiro DE, McSherry GD, Britto P, Cunningham BE, Culnane M, et al. Safety of the maternal-infant zidovudine regimen utilized in the Pediatric AIDS Clinical Trial Group 076 Study. AIDS. 1998;12(14):1805–13. Epub 1998/10/29.

79. Culnane M, Fowler M, Lee SS, McSherry G, Brady M, O'Donnell K, et al. Lack of long-term effects of in utero exposure to zidovudine among uninfected children born to HIV-infected women. Pediatric AIDS Clinical Trials Group Protocol 219/076 Teams. JAMA. 1999;281(2):151–7. Epub 1999/01/23.

80. Hanson IC, Antonelli TA, Sperling RS, Oleske JM, Cooper E, Culnane M, et al. Lack of tumors in infants with perinatal HIV-1 exposure and fetal/neonatal exposure to zidovudine. J Acquir Immune Defic Syndr Hum Retrovirol. 1999;20(5):463–7. Epub 1999/05/04.

81. The Antiretroviral Pregnancy Registry 2013. www.apregistry.com (2013).

82. Tubiana R, Le Chenadec J, Rouzioux C, Mandelbrot L, Hamrene K, Dollfus C, et al. Factors associated with mother-to-child transmission of HIV-1 despite a maternal viral load <500 copies/ml at delivery: a case-control study nested in the French perinatal cohort (EPF-ANRS CO1). Clin Infect Dis. 2010;50(4):585–96. Epub 2010/01/15.

83. European Mode of Delivery Collaboration. Elective caesarean-section versus vaginal delivery in prevention of vertical HIV-1 transmission: a randomised clinical trial. Lancet. 1999;353(9158):1035–9. Epub 1999/04/13.

84. Briand N, Jasseron C, Sibiude J, Azria E, Pollet J, Hammou Y, et al. Cesarean section for HIV-infected women in the combination antiretroviral therapies era, 2000-2010. Am J Obstet Gynecol. 2013;209(4):335.e1–12. Epub 2013/06/25.

85. Reitter A, Stucker A, Linde R, Konigs C, Knecht G, Herrmann E, et al. Pregnancy complications in HIV-positive women: 11-year data from the Frankfurt HIV Cohort. HIV Med. 2014;15(9):525–36. Epub 2014/03/08.

86. Taylor GP, Clayden P, Dhar J, Gandhi K, Gilleece Y, Harding K, et al. British HIV Association guidelines for the management of HIV infection in pregnant women 2012. HIV Med. 2012;13 Suppl 2:87–157. Epub 2012/08/01.

87. Taha TE, Hoover DR, Chen S, Kumwenda NI, Mipando L, Nkanaunena K, et al. Effects of cessation of breastfeeding in HIV-1-exposed, uninfected children in Malawi. Clin Infect Dis. 2011;53(4):388–95. Epub 2011/08/04.

88. Bongain A, Berrebi A, Marine-Barjoan E, Dunais B, Thene M, Pradier C, et al. Changing trends in pregnancy outcome among HIV-infected women between 1985 and 1997 in two southern French university hospitals. Eur J Obstet Gynecol Reprod Biol. 2002;104(2):124–8. Epub 2002/09/11.

89. D'Ubaldo C, Pezzotti P, Rezza G, Branca M, Ippolito G. Association between HIV-1 infection and miscarriage: a retrospective study. DIANAIDS Collaborative Study Group. Diagnosi Iniziale Anomalie Neoplastiche AIDS. AIDS. 1998;12(9):1087–93. Epub 1998/07/14.

90. European Collaborative Study. Pregnancy-related changes in the longer-term management of HIV-infected women in Europe. Eur J Obstet Gynecol Reprod Biol. 2003;111(1):3–8. Epub 2003/10/15.

91. Louis J, Landon MB, Gersnoviez RJ, Leveno KJ, Spong CY, Rouse DJ, et al. Perioperative morbidity and mortality among human immunodeficiency virus infected women undergoing cesarean delivery. Obstet Gynecol. 2007;110(2 Pt 1):385–90. Epub 2007/08/02.

92. Jansen JM, Lijfering WM, Sprenger HG, van der Meer J, van Pampus MG. Venous thromboembolism in HIV-positive women during puerperium: a case series. Blood Coagul Fibrinolysis. 2008;19(1):95–7. Epub 2008/01/09.

93. Fauci AS, Marston HD. Ending AIDS—is an HIV vaccine necessary? N Engl J Med. 2014;370(6):495–8. Epub 2014/02/07.

94. Drake AL, Wagner A, Richardson B, John-Stewart G. Incident HIV during pregnancy and postpartum and risk of mother-to-child HIV transmission: a systematic review and meta-analysis. PLoS Med. 2014;11(2):e1001608. Epub 2014/03/04.

95. ASRM. ASRM Ethics committee report 2010. www.asrm.org/EthicsReports/ (2010).

Chapter 5
The Presence of Hepatitis B and C Virus in Human Gametes and Embryos

Xiao-Ling Hu, Jia-Li You, Hui-Hui Pan, Miao Li, and Yi-Min Zhu

The Presence of HBV in Human Gametes and Embryos

Hepatitis B virus (HBV) infection is a major public health problem worldwide; roughly 30 % of the world's population show serological evidence of current or past infection [1]. Although highly effective vaccines against HBV have been available since 1982, there are still more than 350 million chronic carriers, 75 % of whom reside in the Asia Pacific region. The risk of chronicity varies greatly with the age at which the infection is acquired. For neonates and children younger than 1 year who acquire the infection, the risk of the infection becoming chronic is 90 %. For children aged 1–5 years, the risk is about 30 %, and for children older than 5 years and for adults, the risk according to pooled data decreases to around 2 % [2]. The reason

X.-L. Hu, PhD • J.-L. You, MD • H.-H. Pan, MD • M. Li, MD
Y.-M. Zhu, PhD (✉)
Department of Reproductive Endocrinology, Women's Hospital,
School of Medicine, Zhejiang University, 1 Xueshi Road, Shangcheng,
Hangzhou, Zhejiang 310006, China
e-mail: Xiaolinghu1982@163.com; 21218199@zju.edu.cn; panhuihui2007@qq.com; limiao870219@126.com; zhuyim@zju.edu.cn

© Springer International Publishing Switzerland 2016   119
A. Borini, V. Savasi (eds.), *Assisted Reproductive Technologies and Infectious Diseases*,
DOI 10.1007/978-3-319-30112-9_5

for the high risk of chronicity in neonates and in children younger than 1 year is still uncertain.

About 15–40% patients with chronic hepatitis evolve to liver cirrhosis and hepatocellular carcinoma [3–7]. Approximately 20–30% of patients who are seropositive for HBsAg will transmit the virus to their neonates in the absence of immunoprophylaxis. In women who are HBsAg- and HBeAg-positive, the frequency of transmission increases to 90% [8]. The use of the HBV vaccine and the hepatitis B immunoglobulin in the perinatal stage has effectively prevented most perinatal transmissions of HBV. However, 5–10% of infections still cannot be prevented using these methods [9], and data to explain this phenomenon are lacking. Although hepatotropism is a prominent feature of HBV infection, it is clear that virus is not restricted to any particular organ, but occurs in many extrahepatic tissues, including host somatic cells, oocytes, spermatozoa and embryos [10].

The mechanism of HBV intrauterine infection is not yet clear, but there is a hypothesis that it concerns vertical transmission, in which the sperm, oocyte, or zygote is infected with HBV.

HBV Infection in Semen

In early 1985, Hadchouel et al. [11], using molecular hybridisation, first confirmed the integrated HBV DNA sequences in spermatozoa from two of three patients with HBV infection, suggesting the possibility of true vertical transmission of HBV via the germ line.

Since that time, HBV DNA has continuously been identified in the sperm, either as a free virus in seminal plasma or as an integrated genome in sperm. Wang et al. [12] confirmed the HBV vertical transmission from father to fetus by direct nucleotide sequencing; the homologies of HBV sequences between father and fetus were very high. Using fluorescence in situ hybridisation (FISH), Huang et al. [13] found that the HBV DNA, which integrated into human sperm chromosomes, could create extensively hereditary effects by alteration of the genetic constituent and induction of chromosome aberrations. Moreover, Ali et al. [14] revealed that human sperms carrying HBV genes can pass through the golden hamster oolemma and into the cytoplasm of oocytes and complete fertilisation normally.

After fertilisation, the sperm-mediated HBV genes were able to replicate and their functions were expressed at the mRNA and protein level in early embryonic cells [14]. HBV DNA was also detected in human embryos from three couples (16.7%) with HBsAg-positive men, whereas HBV RNA was detected in embryos from nine couples (69.2%) with HBsAg-positive men [15].

This means that the HBV DNA sequences in infected sperm could be brought into the embryos following fertilisation and the HBV can replicate itself. These studies provided some evidence for the possibility of the vertical transmission of HBV via spermatozoa to the next generation.

It is well known that viral infections and bacteria may be harmful to male fertility [16]. Although Lee et al. [17] report that the sperm concentration and forward motility of semen samples were similar among seropositive and seronegative husbands, after men with azoospermia were excluded. Many studies suggest that HBV infection might also alter sperm parameters [18–21], and decrease sperm motility [19, 22], morphology [17, 22–24] and viability [22, 23]. The higher the viral load, the greater the sperm motility impairment [25].

The molecular mechanism governing the sperm injury is unclear. It may be attributed to increased necrosis or apoptosis of the spermatozoa [19]. Kang et al.'s study [26] showed that HB exposure was not only able to induce reactive oxygen species generation and lipid peroxidation, but also cause apoptosis in sperm cells. At the same time, the mitochondria of the sperm midpiece generate energy to support motility [26]. HBV, through binding to the sperm glycoprotein receptor (ASGP-R), enters into the sperm cell and leads the loss of sperm mitochondrial membrane potential [25]; decreased sperm mitochondrial function may correlate with the diminished motility and reduced fertility [25, 27–29]. The higher the viral load, the greater the sperm motility impairment [25]. Moreover, a persistent inflammatory response induced by HBV may be deleterious to spermatozoa [21].

These studies suggested that HBV infection can do harm to male fertility and create extensive hereditary effects by altering genetic constituents and/or inducing chromosome aberrations, and there is the possibility of the vertical transmission of HBV via the germ line to the next generation.

HBV Infection in Oocytes

The possible vertical transmission of HBV via spermatozoa to embryos has been highlighted by the presence of HBV DNA in spermatozoa. However, the human oocyte is difficult to obtain for research purposes. Previous research has focused on the influence of the perinatal stage of transmission, either in utero or through exposure to blood at or around birth, and few researchers have studied the possibility of vertical transmission by oocyte.

In fact, in 1984, the expression of the HBV genome was detected in the oocytes of two species of amphibians for the first time [30]. Following that, Zhong et al. [31], by analysing HBV nucleotide sequences isolated from three sets of mother/child pairs and finding that the nucleotide and deduced amino acid sequences of the mother and children in two of three families were identical, suggesting the possibility of vertical transmission from mother to children. Animal experience showed that the oocytes can be carriers of HBV, and the HBV DNA sequences could be brought into embryos when the oocytes, with the presence and integration of HBV DNA, were fertilised with normal spermatozoa [14].

In recent years, hepatitis B surface antigen (HBsAg), hepatitis B core antigen (HBcAg), and HBV DNA were detected in ovarian tissues of HBV-infected women [32–34]. These markers were also found in the oocyte [10, 32, 33]. Yu et al. [10] studied the ovarian tissues of 33 pregnant women infected with HBV, which were collected during caesarean section and immunostained for HBsAg; 2 (28 %) were positive for HBsAg in ovarian follicles and the two corresponding infants (100 %) had intrauterine HBV infection.

These results suggest that HBV could infect oocytes and the oocytes infected with HBV might carry a high risk of transmission of HBV to the fetus. However, very few studies have been directly carried out on HBV-infected human oocytes, because the human oocyte is difficult to obtain for research purposes. In recent years there has been a substantial increase in the demand for assisted reproductive technology (ART) in patients infected with HBV infection. Assisted reproductive treatment for such individuals has facilitated the study of the risk of vertical HBV transmission by oocytes. Using FISH, Hu et al. [9] found that HBV DNA was present in 9.6% of oocytes (24 out of 250), the rate of HBV DNA-positive embryos was 13.1% (57 out of 436) among couples in which the woman was HBsAg-seropositive. Nie et al. [15] also detected HBV DNA and HBV RNA in oocytes and embryos from HBsAg-positive women. Thus, HBV may pass through the zona pellucida (ZP) and reach the nuclei and cytoplasm. There seems to be a risk of HBV transmission through oocytes and embryos from HBsAg-positive women.

In Vitro Fertilisation/Intracytoplasmic Sperm Injection Outcomes with HBV-Infected Couples

Since the in vitro fertilisation (IVF) procedure mimics spontaneous conception, the risk of transmitting HBV to the partner and new-born by IVF should be similar for both processes. There is no ethical reason to refuse IVF treatment in HBV-infected patients [24]. In many European centres it is suggested that these patients should be given the opportunity to have children.

Since 95% of patients will seroconvert after vaccination, the best option for couples with one HBsAg-positive partner is the use of HBV vaccination to prevent transmission [8]. However, the main question is that infertility treatment in couples where one or both parents are infected with hepatitis raises many concerns about transmission of the infection to the baby, laboratory technicians, and medical staff, and the contamination of other gametes/embryos that are from virus-free parents in the same laboratory.

Cross-contamination with HBV of five bone marrow samples cryopreserved in liquid nitrogen and the subsequent cross-infection of patients has been clearly demonstrated [35]. Thus, there is no doubt that hepatitis B can survive direct exposure to liquid nitrogen, and under certain conditions result in cross-infection. Consideration of the evidence of liquid nitrogen contamination by HBV, the possibility of contamination or cross-contamination during cryopreservation of gametes and embryos is a realistic possibility. To avoid potential cross-infection, separate storage tanks for

HBV patients are advised. HBV infection has also been reported during artificial insemination and IVF. Berry et al. [36] reported that acute viral hepatitis B in a woman occurred during donor insemination where the donor had not been screened for blood-borne viruses (BBVs) before donation. Widespread contamination during IVF took place in 1991, when 22 human embryos were exposed to HBV in contaminated human serum present in the culture medium. All mothers experienced hepatitis B during the first trimester of pregnancy, and two had hepatitis B surface antigen and HBV DNA at the time of delivery [37].

All contamination occurred before BBV screening was standard. At present, initial screening of couples about to embark on ART treatment is the norm in most fertility clinics worldwide and involves testing for BBVs, including human immunodeficiency virus (HIV), HBV and HCV. This is important from medical, ethical and legal viewpoints. Reproductive care can be targeted to minimise transmission risk to the uninfected partner or future child and to health care staff.

In recent years, there has been a substantial increase in the demand for ART in patients infected with HBV infection. It is not certain whether embryos can become infected at the time of conception or in early pregnancy. Using FISH to visualise the integration of HBV DNA sequences into oocyte and embryo chromosomes of HBV carriers, Hu et al. [9] found that HBV DNA was present in embryos from couples with at least one HBsAg seropositive partner. Rates of HBV DNA-positive embryos were similar among couples in which the woman, man or both partners were HBsAg seropositive, 13.1 % (57 out of 436), 21.3 % (16 out of 75) and 14.9 % (10 out of 67) respectively [9]. Nie et al. [15] showed that HBV DNA and HBV RNA were detected in embryos from couples with HBsAg-positive women or men. These observations provide evidence supporting the hypothesis that the oocyte and sperm might act as a vector for the vertical transmission of HBV to the embryos.

At the same time, the percentage of HBV-positive embryos after intracytoplasmic sperm injection (ICSI) was similar to conventional IVF in male HBV carriers [9, 15]. There is no reason to advise against an ICSI procedure in chronic carriers of HBV.

However, the ICSI procedure bypasses the acrosome reaction and penetration through the ZP—two important mechanisms that protect against sperm-borne pathogens and DNA, and there is no method of selecting sperm without virus infection for ICSI [38]. Another important question is whether infectious particles can be eliminated by sperm processing, so that the healthy female partner can be treated safely. In the past few years, in male HBV patients, sperm-washing has been shown to effectively reduce the risk of vertical transmission and to prevent the introduction of HBV into the oocyte during ICSI. The risk of infected sperm cells acting as vectors in male HBV carriers is not different in IVF compared with ICSI [39]. The pregnancies obtained using ART among couples in which the male partner has chronic viral diseases also produced good obstetric and neonatal results [40]. Although thousands of cycles with the best-practice ART procedures have demonstrated no contamination using sperm from virally infected patients, a viral load in semen can be detected even after sperm-washing procedures [39]. Transmission is possible, both to mothers and newborns, and it is still too early to conclude that these procedures are fully safe. More research to define standardised procedures of sperm-washing specific to each virus and standardised and sensitive methods of viral detection after sperm selection is needed.

Recently, much interest has been focused on the relationship between HBV infection and ART outcome. However, the effect of HBV infection on the outcomes of IVF treatment remains controversial. Lam et al. [41] had compared couples with at least one partner being HBV-seropositive with an HBV seronegative control, and found an improvement in pregnancy and implantation rates after IVF or ICSI for couples where at least one partner is HBV-seropositive. As far as is known, this is the first clinical study that shows the positive effect of male HBV infection on fertilisation. However, it is possible that the results could be attributable to the small sample size. Additional studies with larger samples are required to confirm the results. In contrast to this study, some previous studies suggest possible negative effects of HBV on the results of ART. Despite a comparable response to controlled ovarian hyperstimulation, and similar fertilisation and cleavage rates, couples discordant for HBV or HCV had significantly poorer implantation and pregnancy rates compared with controls: 13 hepatitis B-infected couples (including males and females) were matched with 12 hepatitis C-positive couples and 27 controls [42]. Zhou et al. [23] had compared ICSI and IVF outcomes with HBV-positive and HBV-negative groups, and their finding indicated that HBV infection in men negatively affects the outcome of ICSI cycles, but not IVF cycles. After ICSI and embryo transfer, decreased rates of fertilisation, high-grade embryos, implantation and clinical pregnancy were observed among HBV-positive men compared with matched controls. Oger et al. [21] demonstrated that couples in which male partners have a chronic infection with HBV, have a significantly higher risk of a low fertilisation rate after IVF, which led to a slight decrease in the total number of embryos. Nevertheless, no significant decrease in the pregnancy rates was observed, probably because the low fertilisation rate did not significantly reduce the number of good-quality embryos available for transfer. Furthermore, Shi et al. [24] noted that the duration of infertility was significantly prolonged in HBV-seropositive patients compared with HBV-seronegative patients. Couples with female partners who were HBsAg-seropositive had a significantly lower top-quality embryo rate than the control group. In addition, the fertilisation rates in groups with male or female partners who are HBsAg-seropositive were both significantly lower than for the matched controls. However, there was no significant difference in clinical pregnancy rates between the HBsAg-seropositive and HBsAg-seronegative groups. Ye et al. [43] found that the early abortion rate and the abortion rate with HBV-infected mothers were significantly higher than couples with negative serum HBV markers. The clinical pregnancy rate of the two groups was similar. The increased early abortion rate of pregnancy may be related to HBV-infected embryos. Another two studies did not demonstrate any adverse effect of HBV infection on the assisted reproduction outcomes between the HBV and the control groups. Lee et al. [17] showed that the ongoing pregnancy rate and live-birth rate of couples with both partners being HBsAg positive was not significantly different from couples with discordant HBV serostatus and those couples where both partners were HBsAg-negative.

The authors attributed the unaffected ongoing pregnancy rate to the use of ICSI in couples with low normal sperm morphology (less than 3 %), which may compensate for any defect in fertilisation due to impaired morphology. To assess the impact of male HVB infection on the outcomes of IVF, Bu et al. [44] retrospectively analysed data from 277 subfertile couples undergoing oocyte donation cycles. They found that couples with HBV-seropositive male partners had similar semen parameters, rates of fertilisation, implantation and clinical pregnancy compared with their controls; thus, male HBV infection has little impact on the outcomes of IVF.

The above studies implied that HBV infection might impair gamete and embryo quality. As studies are of smaller sample sizes, and relatively little evidence is available concerning the outcome of this offspring, larger and longer-term follow-up studies still need to assess the impact of HBV infection on gametes, embryos and offspring, and the underlying mechanisms certainly warrant further exploration.

HCV in Oocytes and Embryos

Hepatitis C is a blood-borne liver disease, caused by HCV, which was first identified in 1989. Currently, the worldwide prevalence of HCV infection has reached a figure of 3 %, with 70 % of cases developing chronicity [45]. HCV is a major cause of chronic liver disease in both children and adults worldwide [45]. Eighty percent of HCV infections lead to persistent viraemia [46], and most of patients develop long-term complications, including cirrhosis and liver failure [47, 48]. The rate of progression is highly individual, and some patients have long life expectancies.

Mother-to-child transmission (MTCT) of HCV is one of the several established pathways for HCV transmission. MTCT has become the major route of HCV infection in children [46], affecting up to 10 % of infants born to mothers chronically infected with HCV, but not with HIV [49–53]. It is estimated that 10,000–60,000 newborns worldwide are infected with HCV via MTCT each year [47].

The Effect of HCV Infection

Englert et al. [54] found that HCV-seropositive women had similar embryo quality, implantation, and delivery rates to controls. The effects of HCV infection were essentially confined to ovarian stimulation and follicle maturation. Alterations of granulosa cell function lead to an increased demand for FSH, a lower number of oocytes, and a decreased number of fertilised oocytes; however, once the oocyte is fertilised, the embryos do not appear to be affected and have a similar viability to those of non-infected women. Other researchers have made similar observations in HIV-seropositive women [55]. Furthermore, studies have shown that other viral infections may affect fertility and ovarian function in animals [56, 57]. Englert et al. [54] also found an association between HCV seropositivity and poor ovarian response to stimulation. The authors reported a high number of cancelled cycles resulting from the absence of ovarian response to stimulation in this group of patients and concluded that chronic infection may alter both the reserve of small pre-antral follicles and granulosa cell function. Other researchers' findings confirm those of previous studies that HCV may cause higher cancellation rates of cycles and poor ovarian response in female HCV carriers. HCV infection after MTCT can be persistent [49, 50, 58], and the clinical course varies from asymptomatic, transient hepatitis to chronic hepatitis [59, 60].

Infection with HCV is a newly identified independent risk factor for preterm delivery, perinatal mortality, intrauterine growth restriction, and other complications [61, 62].

The Mechanism for HCV Mother-to-Child Transmission

Mother-to-child transmission of HCV has been reported, but the transmission route is unknown. Its mechanism remains to be elucidated. Both in utero [63] and perinatal [50] transmissions have been proposed. The rate of MTCT from HCV-seropositive and HCV RNA-positive women is 4–6% and transmission occurs almost exclusively from women who are viraemic [46]. Although the timing of transmission is not well defined, it appears that approximately one-third of transmission events occur in utero [48], with the rest occurring peripartum. Risk factors for HCV MTCT include HIV coinfection and intrapartum exposure to maternal blood [46]. Although transmission can be observed with chronic carriers, vertical MTCT appears to be low and occurs mostly during the initial viraemia during pregnancy [64, 65]. Maternal–fetal HCV transmission seems to occur during the perinatal period with fetal exposure to maternal blood and with vaginal secretions at the time of delivery [66].

The risk of transmission of HCV by amniocentesis cannot be established because evidence is lacking. Delamare et al. [67] performed second-trimester amniocentesis on 22 HCV-positive pregnant women, 16 of them being HCV RNA-positive. HCV was detected in a single amniotic fluid sample from a transplacental amniocentesis of a viraemic woman, but the newborn was not infected. Thus, maternal contamination of amniotic fluid cannot be excluded. For years, invasive procedures have been performed without being aware of the serological status of the mother. Nevertheless, all women undergoing an invasive procedure should be tested for HBV, HCV and HIV. Knowledge of the infection is the first necessary step to preventing transmission. If positive, counselling of the parents is needed. In all infections, placental passage during an amniocentesis should be avoided. If an alternative approach is feasible, chorionic villi sampling and cordocentesis should be discouraged. Breastfeeding, HCV genotype, and mode of delivery are not associated with MTCT.

There are very few studies investigating the biology of HCV MTCT, and the reason for the low rate of transmission remains unexplained. The findings that female sex [50] and the absence of HLADR13 in the infant [51] may be risk factors for transmission suggest that the fetal immune system might play a role in protection against and/or facilitation of MTCT.

HCV Infection and Assisted Reproduction Technologies

With proper treatment, some of patients can recover completely [68–70], and some patients infected with HCV would like to have children. Most HCV-serodiscordant couples conceive children naturally, but some are infertile and may seek assisted reproduction Technologies (ARTs).

Assisted reproduction for these patients has been controversial, and the attitudes of IVF centres vary in every country. In addition to the ethical dilemma of offering infertility treatment to these patients, the risk of nosocomial and professional transmission during the highly complex IVF procedure cannot be underestimated [51, 52]. In recent years, there has been a substantial increase in the demand for ART in patients infected with BBV infections such HBV and HCV. We do not yet know if an excess risk of vertical transmission of HCV exists during ART for infertile, infected women.

The use of ART in viraemic women undergoing ART raises questions concerning the safe management of medically assisted procreation for these women and the good practice of oocyte/ embryo cryopreservation and donation. HCV RNA was detected in 89 % of follicular fluid (FF), irrespective of the degree of blood contamination, and in 25 % of the media on day 1. It must be considered that FF is potentially infected. Blood contamination increases the HCV load in the FF. Significantly, rinsing the oocytes seems to discard the HCV RNA. After counselling, attempting IVF in HCV-positive women is justified. Universal guidelines prevent nosocomial infection, and IVF does not specifically increase the professional risk. The mechanism through which HCV infection favours vertical transmission of the virus is still not fully understood. Little information is available about the moment when HCV MTCT occurs, and no procedure has been identified to reduce transmission rates [71].

HCV in Gametes and Embryos

The risk of vertical HCV transmission, or transmission to a woman from an infected man and potentially to gametes or embryos, remains an open question.

Detection of HCV RNA in the semen of infected men is no longer controversial as the problem of false-negative results due to the presence of PCR inhibitors in the ejaculate has been resolved. Numerous studies have demonstrated that sperm preparation, whereby the seminal plasma is removed, reduces the HCV viral load to undetectable levels; none of the recipients became infected [72–74]. HCV has been detected in sperm, but no data are available on FF collected during IVF procedures. Viral contamination of the oocyte before ovulation cannot be excluded, although it is still impossible to demonstrate. Although the presence of HCV in FF has been demonstrated in several studies [75–78], it is unclear whether the viral particles in FF are of an infectious nature, and because HCV culture is difficult to perform in vitro, there are at present no data available to answer this question. Hence, at present it is impossible to evaluate precisely the viral risk presented by FF. Nevertheless, because HCV RNA was detected in most of the follicular aspirates, FF aspirated in HCV-positive women should be considered to have the potential to be infected, irrespective of the degree of macroscopic blood contamination. To evaluate the viral risk induced by ART and to inform the couples, knowledge is required of the localisation of the virus in vivo. FF cannot be collected without follicle rupture, and this may involve a risk of contamination as a result of vascular injury occurring during the ovarian puncture. If HCV penetrates inside the follicle in vivo, its load is likely to be very low and below the viral test threshold. Studies show that active chronic HCV infection does not affect ovarian follicle development despite the detection of HCV RNA in the follicular fluid of 89 % of HCV PCR-positive females, irrespective of the degree of viraemia [77, 78].

Researchers investigating HCV infection and its effects on ovarian follicle development during stimulation for ART reported a higher incidence of apoptosis, which may have a negative impact on pregnancy rates [71, 79–82]. The level of HCV RNA in follicular fluid probably reflects both the circulating HCV RNA load and the degree of blood contamination during retrieval, as suggested by the correlation we found between plasma and FF HCV RNA loads [83]. This is in agreement with Devaux et al. [78], who also reported a significant correlation between HCV serum load and HCV FF load. Some authors related the detection of high HCV RNA levels in the follicular fluid to the vascular injury induced by ovarian puncture [77]. In IVF, the high HCV RNA detection rate in FF (89 %) can most likely be explained by the vessel injuries associated with ovarian puncture. As HCV RNA was detected in 89 % of FF samples, all FF samples should be considered to have the potential to be infected, and consequently the viral risk for retrieved follicles must also be considered.

The possibility of the adsorption of HCV onto granulose cells during ovarian puncture cannot be eliminated. Consequently, HCV present as a result of blood contamination may also be adsorbed onto the granulosa cells, and this may explain the presence of HCV RNA, in spite of the first follicle washing. HCV RNA was never detected in the embryo culture media after washing, removal of granulosa cells and refreshing of the culture media, a result that seems to indicate that HCV RNA might be adsorbed onto granulosa cells in FF during the IVF procedure, although further studies are needed to verify this hypothesis. Furthermore, until implantation the oocytes and embryos are surrounded by the ZP, which is considered to be a physiological protective barrier.

Contamination of the oocytes with HCV remains unknown. Indeed, only a few published studies have examined the risks of contaminating human oocytes or embryos. Oocyte contamination probably occurred during ovarian puncture via the blood and contamination of the FF. Because of the ZP structure, the HCV is probably embedded in the pores of its outer layers. The ability of HCV to pass through the ZP barrier and reach the oocyte cytoplasm or embryonic cells is still unknown.

Hepatitis C virus is associated with unfertilised oocytes surrounded by their intact ZP from anti-HCV antibody-positive. Papaxanthos-Roche et al. [83] report for the first time PCR-detected HCV RNA associated with zona-intact unfertilised human oocytes obtained from HCV RNA-positive women enrolled in an ART programme. In their research the percentage of HCV RNA-positive oocytes was higher after ICSI (85.7 %) than after conventional IVF (64.7 %). This tendency has to be confirmed with a larger number of oocytes, but raises the possibility that microinjection allows viral elements to be transported into the oocyte with the spermatozoon. Indeed, this possibility has been investigated by injecting the oocyte/zygote with a purified solution of viral RNA [84], DNA [85], purified virus solution [86] or contaminated spermatozoa [87]. PCR analysis does not allow one to determine the localisation of the viral RNA; it could be on or in the ZP, in the perivitelline space or inside the oocyte cytoplasm. Washing oocytes or embryos could lower the quantity of virus associated with the ZP, but, as has been demonstrated with bovine viral diarrhoea virus (BVDV), washing and enzymatic treatment (trypsin) did not reliably remove all BVDV that was associated with developed IVF bovine embryos [88, 89]. HCV in the channels of the ZP may be protected from such treatment. Additional research is needed to determine if oocyte washing effectively eliminates HCV. In one study, women were infected with HCV during adulthood and, in light of the absence of serum or supporting cells from oocyte/embryo cultures, oocytes or only their ZP were contaminated, probably by contact with blood during follicular aspiration. However, the ability of HCV to cross cellular compartments was indicated by the analysis of the virus's genome in hepatocytes [90], and by HCV RNA detection in sperm [72–74].

These results suggest the possibility of HCV infecting the oocyte and embryo. Evaluation of the viral risk for oocytes and embryos during IVF has not yet been completely defined, although it cannot be ignored and deserves future study. This procedure may affect IVF outcome by decreasing the number of oocytes for the fertilisation step.

During the IVF procedure, the decreasing HCV RNA titre may be due to a dilution of the virus during the washing of the oocytes, removal of the granulosa cells, and refreshing of the media. It is possible to compare the oocyte washing procedure with a selection procedure using a gradient of Pure Sperm, followed by the washing of spermatozoa, from HCV+ and HIV+ men [91]. Two HCV receptors for HCV have been identified, namely the CD 81 molecule and the low-density lipoprotein receptor [92–95]. The HCV RNA titre was decreased drastically after the selection and washing of spermatozoa from infected men, and preliminary results have confirmed an absence of contamination in both the negative female partner and the newborn [74]. It could therefore be expected that, if the embryo culture media is negative, then the viral risk for the embryos of viraemic women is at least very low and, at most, almost absent.

The present results have shown that thorough rinsing of the oocytes and embryos and refreshing of the media appear to be effective and that, as a consequence, all oocytes could be used. Nonetheless, oocytes that were included in a clot of blood and could not be thoroughly washed must be discarded. Attention must also be paid to the impact of HCV+ genital secretions on the contamination rate of the embryo when the transfer is associated with light cervical bleeding.

Conclusion

For HCV-positive women undergoing ART, more studies are needed to evaluate the risk of HCV contamination to which oocytes/embryos are exposed and to establish good safety guidelines for oocyte/embryo manipulation, cryopreservation and donation. Using serum from an HCV-positive mother for embryo cryopreservation must also be avoided. Consequently, the use of a tested negative serum albumin, or the male partners' serum, is recommended.

References

1. Trépo C, Chan HL, Lok A. Hepatitis B virus infection. Lancet. 2014;384(9959):2053–63. doi:10.1016/S0140-6736(14)60220-8.
2. Lai C, Ratziu V, Yuen M, Poynard T. Viral hepatitis B. Lancet. 2003;362:2089–94.
3. Borgia G, Gentile I. Treating chronic hepatitis B: today and tomorrow. Curr Med Chem. 2006;13(23):2839–55.
4. Coppola N, Marrone A, Pisaturo M, et al. Role of interleukin28-B in the spontaneous and treatment-related clearance of HCV infection in patients with chronic HBV/HCV dual infection. Eur J Clin Microbiol Infect Dis. 2014;33(4):559–67.
5. Coppola N, Potenza N, Pisaturo M, et al. Liver microRNA hsa-miR-125a-5p in HBV chronic infection: correlation with HBV replication and disease progression. PLoS One. 2013;8(7):e65336.
6. Sagnelli E, Stroffolini T, Mele A, et al. Impact of comorbidities on the severity of chronic hepatitis B at presentation. World J Gastroenterol. 2012;18(14):1616–21.

7. Sagnelli E, Stroffolini T, Mele A, Imparato M, Almasio PL, Italian Hospitals' Collaborating Group. Chronic hepatitis B in Italy: new features of an old disease—approaching the universal prevalence of hepatitis B e antigen-negative cases and the eradication of hepatitis D infection. Clin Infect Dis. 2008;46(1):110–3.

8. Practice Committee of American Society for Reproductive Medicine. Hepatitis and reproduction. Fertil Steril. 2008;90(5 Suppl):S226–35.

9. Hu XL, Zhou XP, Qian YL, Wu GY, Ye YH, Zhu YM. The presence and expression of the hepatitis B virus in human oocytes and embryos. Hum Reprod. 2011;26(7):1860–7.

10. Yu M, Jiang Q, Gu X, Ju L, Ji Y, Wu K, Jiang H. Correlation between vertical transmission of hepatitis B virus and the expression of HBsAg in ovarian follicles and placenta. PLoS One. 2013;8(1):e54246.

11. Hadchouel M, Scotto J, Huret JL, Molinie C, Villa E, Degos F, Brechot C. Presence of HBV DNA in spermatozoa: a possible vertical transmission of HBV via the germ line. J Med Virol. 1985;16:61–6.

12. Wang S, Peng G, Li M, Xiao H, Jiang P, Zeng N, Wang Z. Identification of hepatitis B virus vertical transmission from father to fetus by direct sequencing. Southeast Asian J Trop Med Public Health. 2003;34(1):106–13.

13. Huang JM, Huang TH, Qiu HY, Fang XW, Zhuang TG, Qiu JW. Studies on the integration of hepatitis B virus DNA sequence in human sperm chromosomes. Asian J Androl. 2002;4(3):209–12.

14. Ali BA, Huang TH, Xie QD. Detection and expression of hepatitis B virus X gene in one and two-cell embryos from golden hamster oocytes in vitro fertilized with human spermatozoa carrying HBV DNA. Mol Reprod Dev. 2005;70(1):30–6.

15. Nie R, Jin L, Zhang H, Xu B, Chen W, Zhu G. Presence of hepatitis B virus in oocytes and embryos: a risk of hepatitis B virus transmission during in vitro fertilization. Fertil Steril. 2011;95(5):1667–71.

16. Moretti E, Baccetti B, Capitani S, Collodel G. Necrosis in human spermatozoa. II. Ultrastructural features and FISH study in semen from patients with recovered uro-genital infections. J Submicrosc Cytol Pathol. 2005;37(1):93–8.

17. Lee VC, Ng EH, Yeung WS, Ho PC. Impact of positive hepatitis B surface antigen on the outcome of IVF treatment. Reprod Biomed Online. 2010;21(5):712–7.

18. Huret JL, Jeulin C, Hadchouel M, Scotto J, Molinie C. Semen abnormalities in patients with viral hepatitis B. Arch Androl. 1986;17(1):99–100.

19. Moretti E, Federico MG, Giannerini V, Collodel G. Sperm ultrastructure and meiotic segregation in a group of patients with chronic hepatitis B and C. Andrologia. 2008;40(5):286–91.

20. Vicari E, Arcoria D, Di Mauro C, Noto R, Noto Z, La Vignera S. Sperm output in patients with primary infertility and hepatitis B or C virus; negative influence of HBV infection during concomitant varicocele. Minerva Med. 2006;97(1):65–77.

21. Oger P, Yazbeck C, Gervais A, Dorphin B, Gout C, Jacquesson L, Ayel JP, Kahn V, Rougier N. Adverse effects of hepatitis B virus on sperm motility and fertilization ability during IVF. Reprod Biomed Online. 2011;23(2):207–12.

22. Lorusso F, Palmisano M, Chironna M, Vacca M, Masciandaro P, Bassi E, Selvaggi Luigi L, Depalo R. Impact of chronic viral diseases on semen parameters. Andrologia. 2010;42(2):121–6.

23. Zhou XP, Hu XL, Zhu YM, Qu F, Sun SJ, Qian YL. Comparison of semen quality and outcome of assisted reproductive techniques in Chinese men with and without hepatitis B. Asian J Androl. 2011;13(3):465–9.

24. Shi L, Liu S, Zhao W, Zhou H, Ren W, Shi J. Hepatitis B virus infection reduces fertilization ability during in vitro fertilization and embryo transfer. J Med Virol. 2014;86(7):1099–104.

25. Zhou XL, Sun PN, Huang TH, Xie QD, Kang XJ, Liu LM. Effects of hepatitis B virus S protein on human sperm function. Hum Reprod. 2009;24(7):1575–83.

26. Kang X, Xie Q, Zhou X, Li F, Huang J, Liu D, Huang T. Effects of hepatitis B virus S protein exposure on sperm membrane integrity and functions. PLoS One. 2012;7(3):e33471.

27. Marchetti C, Obert G, Deffosez A, Formstecher P, Marchetti P. Study of mitochondrial membrane potential, reactive oxygen species, DNA fragmentation and cell viability by flow cytometry in human sperm. Hum Reprod. 2002;17:1257–65.

28. Piasecka M, Kawiak J. Sperm mitochondria of patients with normal sperm motility and with asthenozoospermia: morphological and functional study. Folia Histochem Cytobiol. 2003;41:125–39.

29. Wang X, Sharma RK, Gupta A, George V, Thomas AJ, Falcone T, Agarwal A. Alterations in mitochondria membrane potential and oxidative stress in infertile men: a prospective observational study. Fertil Steril. 2003;80 Suppl 2:844–50.

30. Lrive-Zerbani A, Gallien CL, Pourcel C. Expression of hepatitis B virus (HBV) genome in the oocytes of two species of amphibians. Biol Cell. 1984;50(3):223–8.

31. Zhong M, Hou J, Luo K. Identification of vertical transmission of hepatitis B virus from mother to children by direct sequencing a segment of surface gene of hepatitis B virus. Zhonghua Yi Xue Za Zhi. 1996;76(3):194–6.

32. Ye F, Yue Y, Li S, Chen T, Bai G, Liu M, Zhang S. Presence of HBsAg, HBcAg, and HBV DNA in ovary and ovum of the patients with chronic hepatitis B virus infection. Am J Obstet Gynecol. 2006;194(2):387–92.

33. Chen LZ, Fan XG, Gao JM. Detection of HBsAg, HBcAg, and HBV DNA in ovarian tissues from patients with HBV infection. World J Gastroenterol. 2005;11(35):5565–7.

34. Lou H, Ding W, Dong M, Zhu Y, Zhou C, Wang Z, Yang X, Yao Q, Li D, Miao M. The presence of hepatitis B surface antigen in the ova of pregnant women and its relationship with intra-uterine infection by hepatitis B virus. J Int Med Res. 2010;38(1):214–9.

35. Tedder RS, Zuckerman MA, Goldstone AH, Hawkins AE, Fielding A, Briggs EM, Irwin D, Blair S, Gorman AM, Patterson KG, Linch DC, Heptonstall J, Brink NS. Hepatitis B transmission from contaminated cryopreservation tank. Lancet. 1995;346(8968):137–40.

36. Berry W, Gottesfeld R, Alter H, Vierling J. Transmission of hepatitis B virus by artificial insemination. JAMA. 1987;257:1079–81.

37. Quint W, Fetter W, van Os H, Heijtink R. Absence of hepatitis B virus (HBV) in children born after exposure of their mothers to HBV during in vitro fertilization. J Clin Microbial. 1994;32:1099–100.

38. Kambin SP, Batzer FR. Assisted reproductive technology in HIV sero-discordant couples. Sex Reprod Menopause. 2004;2:92–100.

39. Garolla A, Pizzol D, Bertoldo A, Menegazzo M, Barzon L, Foresta C. Sperm viral infection and male infertility: focus on HBV, HCV, HIV, HPV, HSV, HCMV, and AAV. J Reprod Immunol. 2013;100(1):20–9.

40. Molina I, Carmen Del Gonzalvo M, Clavero A, Angel López-Ruz M, Mozas J, Pasquau J, Sampedro A, Martínez L, Castilla JA. Assisted reproductive technology and obstetric outcome in couples when the male partner has a chronic viral disease. Int J Fertil Steril. 2014;7(4):291–300.

41. Lam PM, Suen SH, Lao TT, Cheung LP, Leung TY, Haines C. Hepatitis B infection and outcomes of in vitro fertilization and embryo transfer treatment. Fertil Steril. 2010;93(2):480–5.

42. Pirwany IR, Phillips S, Kelly S, Buckett W, Tan SL. Reproductive performance of couples discordant for hepatitis B and C following IVF treatment. J Assist Reprod Genet. 2004;21(5):157–61.

43. Ye F, Liu Y, Jin Y, Shi J, Yang X, Liu X, Zhang X, Lin S, Kong Y, Zhang L. The effect of hepatitis B virus infected embryos on pregnancy outcome. Eur J Obstet Gynecol Reprod Biol. 2014;172:10–4.
44. Bu Z, Kong H, Li J, Wang F, Guo Y, Su Y, Zhai J, Sun Y. Effect of male hepatitis B virus infection on outcomes of in vitro fertilization and embryo transfer treatment: insights from couples undergoing oocyte donation. Int J Clin Exp Med. 2014;7(7):1860–6.
45. Pearlman BL. Hepatitis C, infection: a clinical review. South Med J. 2004;97:364–73.
46. Smyk-Pearson S, Tester I, Klarquist J, Palmer B, Pawlotsky J, et al. Functional suppression by FoxP3+CD4+CD25high regulatory T cells during acute hepatitis C virus infection. J Infect Dis. 2008;197:46–57.
47. Golden-Mason L, Rosen HR. Natural killer cells: primary target for hepatitis C virus immune evasion strategies? Liver Transpl. 2006;12:363–72.
48. Iorio R, Giannattasio A, Sepe A, Terracciano LM, Vecchione R, et al. Chronic hepatitis C in childhood: an 18-year experience. Clin Infect Dis. 2005;41:1431–7.
49. Nagata I, Iizuka T, Harada Y, Okada T, Matsuda R, Tanaka Y, Tanimoto K, Shiraki K. Prospective study of mother-to-infant transmission of hepatitis C virus. In: Nishioka K, Suzuki H, Mishiro S, Oda T, editors. Viral hepatitis and liver disease. Tokyo: Springer; 1994. p. 468–70.
50. Ohto H, Terazawa S, Sasaki N, Sasaki N, Hino K, Ishiwata C, Kako M, Ujiie N, Endo C, Matsui A, Okamoto H, Mishiro S. The Vertical Transmission of Hepatitis C Virus Collaborative Study Group. Transmission of hepatitis C virus from mothers to infants. N Engl J Med. 1994;330:744–50.
51. Chang MH. Mother-to-infant transmission of hepatitis C virus. Clin Invest Med. 1996;19:368–72.
52. Spencer JD, Latt N, Beeby PJ, Collins E, Saunders JB, McCaughan GW, Cossart YE. Transmission of hepatitis C virus to infants of human immunodeficiency virus-negative intravenous drug-using mothers: rate of infection and assessment of risk factors for transmission. J Viral Hepat. 1997;4:395–409.
53. Thomas DL. Mother-infant hepatitis C transmission: second generation research. Hepatology. 1999;29:992–3.
54. Englert Y, Moens E, Vannin AS, Liesnard C, Emiliani S, Delbaere A, Devreker F. Impaired ovarian stimulation during in vitro fertilization in women who are seropositive for hepatitis C virus and seronegative for human immunodeficiency virus. Fertil Steril. 2007;88:607–11.

55. Englert Y, Lesage B, Van Vooren JP, Liesnard C, Place I, Vannin AS, et al. Medically assisted reproduction in the presence of chronic viral diseases. Hum Reprod Update. 2004;10:149–62.
56. Fray MD, Paton DJ, Alenius S. The effects of bovine viral diarrhea virus on cattle reproduction in relation to disease control. Anim Reprod Sci. 2000;60:615–27.
57. Fray MD, Mann GE, Clarke MC, Charleston B. Bovine viral diarrhoea virus: its effect on ovarian function in the cow. Vet Microbiol. 2000;77:185–94.
58. Nagata I, Shiraki K, Tanimoto K, Harada Y, Tanaka Y, Okada T. Mother-to-infant transmission of hepatitis C virus. J Pediatr. 1992;120:432–4.
59. Zanetti AR, Tanzi E, Paccagnini S, Principi N, Pizzocolo G, Caccamo ML, D'Amico E, Cambie G, Vecchi L. Mother-to-infant transmission of hepatitis C virus. Lombardy Study Group on Vertical HCV Transmission. Lancet. 1995;345:289–91.
60. Palomba E, Manzini P, Fiammengo P, Maderni P, Saracco G, Tovo PA. Natural history of perinatal hepatitis C virus infection. Clin Infect Dis. 1996;23:47–50.
61. Japanese Red Cross Non-A Non-B Hepatitis Research Group. Effect of screening hepatitis C virus antibody and hepatitis B virus core antibody on incidence of post transfusion hepatitis. Lancet. 1991;338:1040–1.
62. Kato N, Sekiya H, Ootsuyama Y, Nakazawa T, Hijikata M, Ohkoshi S, Shimotohno K. Humoral immuno response to hypervariable region 1 of the putative envelope glycoprotein (gp70) of hepatitis C virus. J Virol. 1993;67:3923–30.
63. Weiner AJ, Thaler MM, Crawford K, Ching K, Kansopon J, Chien DY, Hall JE, Hu F, Houghton M. A unique, predominant hepatitis C virus variant found in an infant born to a mother with multiple variants. J Virol. 1993;67:4365–8.
64. Van der Poel CL, Ebeling F. Hepatitis C virus: epidemiology, transmission and prevention. Curr Stud Hematol Blood Transf Basel. 1998;62:208–36.
65. Michielsen PP, Van Damme P. Viral hepatitis and pregnancy. Acta Gastroenterol Belg. 1999;62:21–9.
66. Poiraud S, Cohen J, Amiot X, Berkane N, et al. Étude cas-témoin des facteurs de risque de transmission materno-infantile du virus de l'hépatite C (VHC). Gastroenterol Clin Biol. 2001;25:A96.
67. Delamare C, Carbonne B, Heim N, Berkane N, Petit JC, Uzan S, Grange JD. Detection of hepatitis C virus RNA (HCV RNA) in amniotic fluid: a prospective study. J Hepatol. 1999;31:416–20.

68. Roudot-Thoraval F, Bastie A, Pawlotsky JM, Dhumeaux D. Epidemiological factors affecting the severity of hepatitis C virus-related liver disease: a French survey of 6,664 patients. The Study Group for the Prevalence and the Epidemiology of Hepatitis C Virus. Hepatology. 1997;26:485–90.

69. Halfon P, Riflet H, Renou C, Quentin Y, Cacoub P. Molecular evidence of male-to-female sexual transmission of hepatitis C virus after vaginal and anal intercourse. J Clin Microbiol. 2001;39:1204–6.

70. Thomas DL, Seeff LB. Natural history of hepatitis C. Clin Liver Dis. 2005;9:383–98.

71. Izuma M, Kobayashi K, Shiina M, Ueno Y, Ishii M, Shimosegawa T, Toyota T, Kakimi K, Miyazawa M. In vitro cytokine production of peripheral blood mononuclear cells in response to HCV core antigen stimulation during interferon-beta treatment and its relevance to sCD8 and sCD30. Hepatol Res. 2000;18:218–29.

72. Levy R, Tardy JC, Bourlet T, Cordonier H, Mion F, Lornage J, Guerin JF. Transmission risk of hepatitis C virus in assisted reproductive techniques. Hum Reprod. 2000;15:810–6.

73. Leruez-Ville M, Kunstmann JM, De Almeida M, Rouzioux C, Chaix ML. Detection of hepatitis C virus in the semen of infected men. Lancet. 2000;356:42.

74. Cassuto NG, Sifer C, Feldmann G, Bouret D, Moret F, Benifla JL, Porcher R, Naouri M, Neuraz A, Alvarez S, et al. A modified RT-PCR technique to screen for viral RNA in the semen of hepatitis C virus-positive men. Hum Reprod. 2002;17:3153–6.

75. Papaxanthos-Roche A, Trimoulet P, Hocké C, Fleury HJA, Mayer G. Detection of HCV RNA in follicular fluid. In: First congress on obstetrics gynecology and infertility. 1999; p. 28–31

76. Leruez-Ville M, Cohen-Bacrie P, Selva J, Chaix ML, Bergére M, Rouzioux C, Plachot M. Le virus de l'hépatite C dans les liquides de ponctions folliculaires des femmes infectées. Reprod Hum Horm. 2001;6:385–90.

77. Sifer C, Benifla JL, Branger M, Devaux A, Brun-Vezinet F, Madelenat P, Feldmann G. Effects of hepatitis C virus on the apoptosis percentage of granulosa cells in vivo in women undergoing IVF: preliminary results. Hum Reprod. 2002;17:1773–6.

78. Devaux A, Soula V, Sifer C, Branger M, Naouri M, Porcher R, Poncelet C, Neuraz A, Alvarez S, Benifla JL, et al. Hepatitis C virus detection in follicular fluid and culture media from HCV+ women, and viral risk during IVF procedures. Hum Reprod. 2003;18:2342–9.

79. Oosterhuis GJ, Michgelsen HW, Lambalk CB, Schoemaker J, Vermes I. Apoptotic cell death in human granulosa-lutein cells: a possible

indicator of in vitro fertilization outcome. Fertil Steril. 1998;70:747–9.

80. Hahn CS, Cho YG, Kang BS, Lester IM, Hahn YS. The HCV core protein acts as a positive regulator of fas-mediated apoptosis in a human lymphoblastoid T cell line. Virology. 2000;276:127–37.

81. Piazzolla G, Tortorella C, Schiraldi O, Antonaci S. Relationship between interferon-gamma, interleukin-10, and interleukin-12 production in chronic hepatitis C and in vitro effects of interferon-alpha. J Clin Immunol. 2000;20:54–61.

82. Taya N, Torimoto Y, Shindo M, Hirai K, Hasebe C, Kohgo Y. Fas-mediated apoptosis of peripheral blood mononuclear cells in patients with hepatitis C. Br J Haematol. 2000;110:89–97.

83. Papaxanthos-Roche A. PCR-detected hepatitis C virus RNA associated with human zona-intact oocytes collected from infected women for ART. Hum Reprod. 2004;19(5):1170–5.

84. Gamarnik AV, Boddeker N, Andino R. Translation and replication of human rhinovirus type 14 and mengovirus in Xenopus oocytes. J Virol. 2000;74:11983–7.

85. Baskar JF, Furnari B, Huang ES. Demonstration of developmental anomalies in mouse fetuses by transfer of murine cytomegalovirus DNA injected eggs to surrogate mothers. J Infect Dis. 1993;167:1288–95.

86. Tebourdi L, Testart J, Cerutti I, Moussu JP, Loeuillet A, Courtot AM. Failure to infect embryos after virus injection in mouse zygotes. Hum Reprod. 2002;17:760–4.

87. Chan AWS, Luetjens CM, Dominko T, Ramalho-Santos J, Simerly CR, Hewitson L, Schatten G. Foreign DNA transmission by ICSI: injection of spermatozoa bound with exogenous DNA results in embryonic GPF expression and live Rhesus monkey births. Mol Hum Reprod. 2000;6:26–33.

88. Bielanski A, Jordan L. Washing or washing and trypsin treatment is ineffective for removal of noncytopathic bovine viral diarrhea virus from bovine oocytes or embryos after experimental viral contamination of an in vitro fertilization system. Theriogenology. 1996;46:1467–76.

89. Trachte EA, Stringfellow DA, Riddell KP, Galik PK, Riddell MG, Wright JC. Washing and trypsin treatment of in vitro-derived bovine embryos exposed to bovine viral diarrhea virus. Theriogenology. 1998;50:717–26.

90. Shimizu YK, Igarashi H, Kanematu T, Fujiwara K, Wong DC, Purcell RH, Yoshikura H. Sequence analysis of the hepatitis C virus genome recovered from serum, liver, and peripheral blood mononuclear cells of infected chimpanzees. J Virol. 1997;71:5769–73.

91. Bourlet T, Levy R, Laporte S, Blachier S, Bocket L, et al. Multicenter quality control for the detection of hepatitis C Virus RNA in seminal plasma specimens. J Clin Microbiol. 2003;41(2):789–93.

92. Pileri P, Uematsu Y, Campagnoli S, Galli G, Falugi F, Petracca R. Binding of hepatitis C virus to CD81. Science. 1998;282:938–41.

93. Flint M, Maidens C, Loomis-Price L, Shotton C, Dubuisson J, Monk P. Characterisation of hepatitis C virus E2 glycoprotein interaction with a putative cellular receptor CD 81. J Virol. 1999;73:6235–44.

94. Germi R, Crance JM, Garin D, Zarski JP, Drouet E. Les récepteurs du virus de l'Hépatite C données actuelles. Gastroenterol Clin Biol. 2001;25:1011–5.

95. LaVoie HA, Garmey JC, Day RN, Veldhuis JD. Concerted regulation of low density lipoprotein receptor gene expression by follicle-stimulating hormone and insulin-like growth factor I in porcine granulosa cells: promoter activation, messenger ribonucleic acid stability, and sterol feedback. Endocrinology. 1999;140:178–86.

Chapter 6

Detection of Hepatitis C Virus in the Semen of Infected Men and Reproductive Assistance in HCV Discordant Couples: An Overview

Valeria Savasi and Luca Mandia

Epidemiology of Hepatitis C Virus Infection

Hepatitis C virus (HCV) is a single-stranded RNA member of the *Flaviviridae* family. The virus has an extraordinary heterogeneity owing to its lack of ability to correct copying errors made during viral replication. Many of its nucleotide changes result in a non-functional genome or a replication-incompetent virus (lethal mutants), whereas others persist and account for the incredible viral diversity. Viral heterogeneity takes several forms depending upon the degree of diversity, such as quasispecies (families of different, but highly similar, strains that develop within an infected host over time, with a nucleotide sequence homology greater than 95 %) and over decades and centuries, the degree of HCV diversity

_____

V. Savasi, MD, PhD (✉)
Unit of Obstetrics and Gynecology, Department of Biomedical
and Clinical Sciences, Hospital "L. Sacco", University of Milan, Milan, Italy
e-mail: valeria.savasi@unimi.it

L. Mandia, MD, PhD
Department of Gynecology and Obstetrics, University of Milan, Milan, Italy

© Springer International Publishing Switzerland 2016   143
A. Borini, V. Savasi (eds.), *Assisted Reproductive
Technologies and Infectious Diseases*,
DOI 10.1007/978-3-319-30112-9_6

has evolved into several distinct genotypes of the virus. Sequence homology among the genotypes is less than 80%.

There are six genotypes and numerous subtypes of HCV. Globally, genotype 1 is the most common, accounting for 46% of all infections; followed by genotypes 3 (22%), and genotypes 2 and 4 (13% each). Subtype 1b accounted for 22% of all infections at the global level. There were significant variations across regions, with genotype 1 dominating in Australasia, Europe, Latin America and North America (53–71% of all cases) and genotype 3 accounting for 40% of all infections in Asia. Genotype 4 was most common (71%) in North Africa and the Middle East, but when Egypt was excluded, it accounted for 34%, whereas genotype 1 accounted for 46% of infections across the same region. This heterogeneity is extremely important in the diagnosis of infection, pathogenesis of disease, and the response to treatment; it prevents the development of conventional vaccines, allows the virus to escape eradication by the host's immune system, and affects the completeness of the response to antiviral therapies.

The virus has developed numerous strategies to impair immune responses and evade the host immune system, by delaying and reducing both the intrinsic and adaptive immune response arms. All these characteristics determine a great ability to establish a chronic infection, usually without producing striking symptoms, until the emergence of long-term complications, such as hepatic fibrosis, cirrhosis and hepatocellular carcinoma.

With the advent of new antivirals, HCV infection could in theory be curable in nearly all patients, and with focused strategies to screen and cure current infections in addition to preventing new HCV cases, the number of infections can be significantly lowered or eliminated within the next 15–20 years.

The just published "*Global epidemiology and genotype distribution of the hepatitis C virus infection*" [1] report includes data for anti-HCV prevalence from 87 countries—accounting for 88% of the world's adult population and 84% of the estimated global anti-HCV population—and HCV viraemic rates for 54 countries—accounting for 77% of the world's adult population and 73% of the estimated viraemic HCV population—the global prevalence of anti-HCV was estimated at 2.0% (1.7–2.3%) among adults and

1.6 % (1.3–2.1 %) for all ages, corresponding to 104 (87–124) million and 115 (92–149) million infections respectively. The viraemic prevalence was 1.4 % (1.2–1.7 %) among adults and 1.1 % (0.9–1.4 %) in all ages corresponding to 75 (62–89) million and 80 (64–103) respectively.

About one quarter of human immunodeficiency virus (HIV)-infected persons in the United States are also infected with HCV (CDC Data). Thus, coinfection with HIV and HCV is common (50–90 %) among HIV-infected injection drug users (IDUs). The seroprevalence of anti-HCV is increased among promiscuous heterosexuals and men who have sex with men (MSM). HCV infection is often prevalent among HIV-infected populations, with one-third of HIV-infected Americans, and seven million worldwide being coinfected. Chronic HCV infection is now the leading cause of death, after AIDS-related complications, among HIV-infected individuals in areas where highly active antiretroviral therapy (HAART) is available. HIV coinfection exacerbates HCV disease, increasing the likelihood of cirrhosis and HCV-related mortality. The prevalence of HCV coinfection varies, depending on the mode of HIV transmission [2].

Transmission of Hepatitis C Virus

The transmission of HCV is a complex issue. HCV is transmitted mainly through percutaneous exposure to blood (transfusions, transplants), needle sticks, or the contamination of supplies shared among haemodialysis patients or intravenous drug abusers. Although most patients infected with HCV in the USA and Europe acquired the disease through intravenous drug use or blood transfusion, nowadays, very rare, non-identifiable risk factors for HCV infection can be hypothesized in cases with new infections. A potential mechanism of transmission in these instances is mucosal exposure to infectious blood or to body fluids containing blood, or inapparent percutaneous exposure through personal hygiene items (e.g. shared razors or toothbrushes). Then, in many situations, it is difficult to rule out the possibility that transmission resulted from common exposure to risk factors other than sexual exposure [3]. HCV RNA has also been detected in menstrual fluid and semen and both sexual and vertical transmissions have been suggested as alternative modes of transmission of HCV.

Epidemiological studies evaluated HCV sexual transmission. To our knowledge, three prospective cohort studies of monogamous heterosexual couples have been published [4–6]. The HCV Partners' study published in 2013 followed 500 monogamous heterosexual couples to provide quantifiable risk information for counselling long-term monogamous heterosexual couples in which one partner has a chronic HCV infection [5]. Criteria for study participation by each couple included having a heterosexual relationship for a minimum of 36 months, being monogamous for the duration of the relationship as reported by both partners and a minimum of three sexual contacts by the couple in the preceding 6 months. Couples were excluded if either partner had known HIV or hepatitis B virus (HBV) infection, had undergone previous organ transplantation, or was currently using antiviral or immunosuppressive therapy, or if both partners reported a history of IDU. Couples were interviewed separately for lifetime risk factors for HCV infection, within-couple sexual practices, and the sharing of personal grooming items. The median duration of the couples' sexual relationships was 15 years (range, 2–52 years). Among the 500 partners of anti-HCV-positive index subjects, 20 (4%) were confirmed to be anti-HCV-positive and 13 of the 20 partners were HCV RNA-positive. HCV genotyping/subtyping and HCV serotyping confirmed nine couples to be concordant, eight couples to be discordant and three couples to be of indeterminate status. Of the + genotype-concordant couples, both partners of six couples were viraemic, allowing phylogenetic analyses, showing that although the overall prevalence of HCV infection among the partners of anti-HCV-positive index subjects was 20 out of 500 (4%), the prevalence of HCV infection among partners potentially attributable to sexual contact was 3 out of 500 (0.6%; 95% CI, 0.0–1.3%) Based on 8377 person-years of follow-up, the maximum incidence rate of HCV transmission by sex was 0.07% per year (95% confidence interval, 0.01–0.13) or approximately 1 per

190,000 sexual contacts. No specific sexual practices were related to HCV positivity among couples.

Other authors suggest caution as the efficiency of HCV transmission by sexual intercourse is generally very low, but some studies showed an increase risk related to particular sexual practices, such as unprotected anal intercourse and vaginal intercourse during menstruation. Another large, prospective study included 895 monogamous, heterosexual partners of HCV-infected individuals who were followed for 10 years. The average weekly rate of sexual intercourse was 1.8. All couples denied practicing anal intercourse, having sex during menstruation, or using condoms. During follow-up, three patients developed HCV infection; however, molecular analysis showed that none had acquired it from their spouse. This risk seems to be related to the number of incidents of sexual intercourse [6].

The CDC Guidelines published in 2010 report that the sexual transmission of HCV has been considered to occur rarely, but CDC surveillance data indicate that 10 % of patients with acute HCV infection report having had contact with a known HCV-infected sexual partner as the only risk of infection (www.cdc.gov/std/treatment/2010/hepC.htm). Patients with acute or chronic HCV infection should be advised that transmission via sexual or household contacts is a possibility, although the risk is relatively low. It is likely that the use of condoms lowers the risk of sexual transmission further, similar to HBV and HIV. However, the United States Public Health Service and a consensus statement issued by the National Institutes of Health have not recommended barrier precautions between stable monogamous sexual partners.

Detection of Hepatitis C Virus in the Semen of Infected Men and Reproductive Assistance in HCV-Discordant Couples

During the past few years, assisted reproduction has been facing a new demand from patients requiring assisted reproductive technology (ART): couples at risk of partner-to-partner viral infection and mother-to-child transmission of viral infections—mainly HIV-1,

HCV and HIV–HCV co-infected partners. The request for reproductive assistance in this context has been mainly for two medical
reasons: either to overcome an infertility problem or to decrease
the risk of horizontal transmission. This is directly correlated with
three different scenarios: both partners being infected, female-only
infection and male-only infection. The primary goal of assisting
discordant couples is to protect the uninfected man or woman from
viral horizontal transmission and consequently remove the risk of
vertical transmission if the mother is unaffected. Also, in assisted
reproduction, HCV transmission may pose a risk for the newborn,
for gametes or embryos from non-contaminated parents and also
for technicians.

   The debate on HCV-discordant couples requiring assisted reproduction is still open today. As most of the HCV patients enrolled in
ART programmes are coinfected with HIV, in this scenario, coinfection is a crucial point when dealing with the sexual transmission
of HCV, as the latter seems to be more frequent in patients coinfected by HIV, as shown by Filippini et al. [7] and Briat et al. [8].

   The presence of the virus in the sperm is not a controversial
issue. Several studies have analysed semen samples of HCV-
positive men to define the possible presence of HCV RNA in
semen fractions with controversial results. The majority of the
papers published in the literature reported a prevalence of seminal
HCV RNA varying from 0 to 30 % using different PCR techniques.
These contradictory findings can be explained by differences in the
collection and/or storage of samples and in the sensitivity of the
assays designed to detect HCV RNA. An additional critical point
is that HCV viral loads in seminal plasma show dramatic and rapid
variations through time. Anyway, today we can assert that viral
particles may be found in seminal plasma and in the other cell fractions, but not in spermatozoa [9].

   The study by Briat et al. [8] included 120 HCV-positive men, 82
of them coinfected with HIV-1, and demonstrated that HCV RNA
was more frequently found in the semen of men coinfected with
HIV-1 (37.8% in men coinfected with HIV-1vs 18.4% in those with
only HCV infection).

   The presence of the HIV virus in semen could therefore be a
bias for the presence of HCV. However, other studies [10] reported

that HIV-positive status does not influence the presence of HCV RNA in the semen, and inversely, the presence of HIV RNA in the seminal plasma is not influenced by the HCV status. Only one paper by Bourlet et al. in 2009 [11] reported a 4-year follow-up French multicentre study that enrolled 86 HCV-serodiscordant couples. All the men enrolled were chronically infected by HCV and 10 of them by HIV. From the 58 couples effectively enrolled in the ART programmes of various reproductive centres, 24 pregnancies and 28 newborns were achieved. All of them tested negative for HCV RNA in blood.

Our group conducted a prospective study to assess prospectively the viral risk for HCV-discordant couples in an ART programme with the aims:

1. To report the clinical results of reproductive assistance in a cohort of HCV-discordant couples treated all in the same centre
2. To evaluate the serological status of mothers and babies
3. To open the discussion of whether or not infertile HCV couples should be treated as infected couples. Between January 2008 and December 2010 in our Reproductive Centre at Sacco Hospital, University of Milan, we enrolled 35 couples with a seropositive HCV male and seronegative partner undergoing assisted reproduction. The ART laboratory we used for the procedure is considered a "viral risk" area, separated from laboratory facilities used for couples negative for HIV, HBV and HCV. Specific precautions were implemented against the risk of HIV, HCV and HBV contamination, as recommended by the French decree of 10 May 2001 [12], and the potentially infected gametes and embryos were handled separately. A special biosafety cabinet workstation was used for all tasks that involved handling sperm, oocytes and embryos.

All couples completed the immuno-virological and fertility triage, and were treated according to our protocols. Couples were advised to use a condom during intercourse throughout the period of the ART programme. After sperm collection we performed "sperm-washing" to separate motile spermatozoa from non-sperm cells, immotile spermatozoa and seminal plasma. After swim-up, a supernatant volume of 500 µl was recovered and used for intrauterine insemination (IUI) or intracytoplasmic sperm injection (ICSI) ovulation induction using gonadotrophins. We simultaneously performed an HCV assay for the qualitative and quantitative detection of HCV RNA in male blood plasma, but we decided to not perform PCR to detect HCV RNA in the final swim-up after sperm-washing, because previous papers have demonstrated that the HCV virus is not able to infect spermatozoa after swim-up. The status of the female partner was confirmed by HCV antibody testing measurements during the 2 weeks before each ART attempt. These tests were repeated 6 months after treatment and again at delivery for pregnant women. The children born were tested once after birth for HCV RNA and after 18 months to check HCV antibodies.

The risk factors for HCV infection were intravenous drug usage in 4 (11%), blood transfusion in 1 (3%) and undetermined in 30 (86%). The range of viral load for HCV was between 1742 and 360911 million of copies/ml in blood plasma. None of the males had ever received any treatment with antiviral drugs. Infertility was originally in the female or male in 29% or 71% of the cases respectively. The main cause of female infertility was fallopian tube occlusion (10 patients) and the main cause of male infertility was abnormal semen parameters. None of the seminal samples analysed in our study had normal values in all seminal parameters (number, motility, morphology), but the role of HCV in male infertility is still to be defined. Bourlet et al. [11, 13] and Garrido et al. [14] supported the findings that HCV does not influence male infertility. In disagreement with Bourlet, who mainly performed ICSI in his study because of the use of frozen–thawed semen, we performed either IUI or ICSI on the unique basis of the infertility problems of the couples.

Fourteen couples underwent superovulation and IUI. The mean age (±SD) was 38±4 for female partners. Basal FSH in women was 6.9±2.9 IU/l. Couples had a mean of three treatments. Seventy per cent of pregnancies were obtained in the first three attempts. Twenty-one couples were treated using second-level ART procedures (mean number of cycles per couple 1.8). The mean age was (±SD) 37±3 for female partners. The pregnancy rate in the IUI group (15%) is higher than the rate reported for infertile couples by the Italian National register, which collects the ART data from all Italian infertility centres (11 %). This difference is reasonably due to the small number of procedures (47 IUIs) performed. The pregnancy rate for ICSI was 18 % and the mean age of the women was 38 years. The Italian National register and Bourlet et al. [11] reported similar pregnancy rates in uninfected infertile couples. The fertilisation rate was high (88 %), supporting the hypothesis that the spermatozoa of HCV-infected patients might be competent. The pregnancy outcome of all the babies was good, with no preterm labour.

It is currently unclear why HCV should be less transmissible than HIV by sexual contact, similar in frequency for vertical trans-mission, and probably more infectious through parenteral expo-sure. It has been argued that the low infectivity of HCV by sexual contact is related to its low titre in genital secretions, but titres of free HIV are also low. It is possible that the presence of HIV-infected lymphocytes might be more relevant for the transmission of HIV. However, interesting data by Azzari et al. [15] show that maternal peripheral blood mononuclear cell culture (PBMNC) infection by HCV and viral replicative activity in PBMNCs are important factors in the transmission of HCV from mother to child. It has been suggested that HCV might infect not only hepatocytes, but also mononuclear lymphocytes, including B cells that express the CD81 molecule, a putative HCV receptor. Thus, HCV is able to enter into lymphocytes and replicate itself, as demonstrated by the presence of a negative strain of HCV RNA, a marker of its replication. The role of PBMNC infection by HCV is controver-sial, but it has been demonstrated that lymphocytes may act as an HCV reservoir and play a key role in the relapse of HCV disease after liver transplantation [8] or after the discontinuation of inter-feron therapy. Only one author has analysed the quasispecies of the virus in blood and semen and did not find any differences [8]. The author observed that some men with a low blood viral load had detectable HCV RNA in their semen and conversely some men with a high blood viral load did not . Such discrepancies could be explained by local replication in leukocytes of the male genital tract, as reported in blood lymphocytes and monocytes [16–18]. Anyway, phylogenetic comparison of HCV quasispecies in blood and in semen showed no evidence of HCV replication in genital leukocytes; however, a phylogenetic structure was observed between compartments and Briat et al. [8] suggested that HCV particles in semen might originate from passive passage from the blood, with preferential transfer of some variants.

There is also an additional risk to consider. The risk of HCV transmission during reproductive procedures is not documented and there is only a prospective multicentre paper reporting assisted reproduction in 56 HCV-serodiscordant couples. The aim of this study was to evaluate if the sperm-washing method was able to reduce levels of HCV in semen and the risk of HCV transmission to the newborn [11]. It is open to discussion whether or not infertile HCV-discordant couples should be treated as infected couples, and whether it is necessary to apply specific laboratory precautions. Since the publication of a case report that described the transmission of HCV from an infected patient undergoing IVF to two non-infected patients undergoing IVF within the same clinic during the same time period (ASRM), there is great concern among clinicians. Although data on laboratory/nosocomial transmission of HCV during assisted reproduction are both limited and controversial, showing that transmission of viral hepatitis in assisted reproduction is possible, but with a risk of unknown magnitude, it is necessary for infertile HCV-discordant couples to be included in protocols of controlled assisted reproduction procedures to avoid any risk of HCV transmission to the partner and to the staff preparing the sample, and laboratory contamination of the gametes of other non-infected couples through cryopreservation and manipulation [22].

Indeed, in assisted reproduction HCV transmission raises some questions. One of these is that specific guidelines establishing the behaviour of physicians in reproductive medicine have not yet been established. Should we treat HCV-discordant couples who require reproductive assistance? Most researchers believe that a sequential preparation with density–gradient centrifugation–washing–swim-up is recommended for HCV-positive men, similar to HIV semen preparation [11, 19, 20]. Other authors do not consider HCV to be a sexually transmitted disease and for this reason believe that it is unnecessary to perform sperm-washing (http://www.sginf.ch). The second main question is: should fertile HCV-discordant couples be treated? We believe that it is not necessary if they do not need reproductive assistance.

Conclusion

We believe that even if sexual transmission of HCV is very low, in subfertile or infertile couples, sperm-washing should be used to treat HCV-positive semen before ART. We suggest that it might not be necessary to perform nested PCR to detect HCV RNA in the final pellet, as suggested by Bourlet et al. and presently required by French legislation [11]. As the presence of HCV in semen implies a possible risk of nosocomial contamination, safety regulations must be strictly applied in assisted reproduction laboratories. As reported by Englert et al. [21] it seems to be "safer and more ethically acceptable to handle patients with the same levels of risk together, i.e. detected viral carriers in one laboratory, negatively screened patients in another, rather than to mix patients with clearly different risk levels". Therefore, the laboratory used for ART should be a "viral risk" area separated from the laboratory used for couples negative for HIV, HBV, HCV. International guidelines should be developed through studies on larger populations of chronically HCV-infected individuals.

References

1. Gower E, Estes C, Blach S, Razavi-Shearer K, Razavi H. Global epidemiology and genotype distribution of the hepatitis C virus infection. J Hepatol. 2014;61(1 Suppl):S45–57.
2. Taylor LE, Swan T, Mayer KH. HIV coinfection with hepatitis C virus: evolving epidemiology and treatment paradigms. Clin Infect Dis. 2012;55 Suppl 1:S33–42.
3. Zylberberg H, Thiers V, Lagorce D, Squadrito G, Leone F, Berthelot P, Bréchot C, Pol S. Epidemiological and virological analysis of couples infected with hepatitis C virus. Gut. 1999;45(1):112.

4. Tahan V, Karaca C, Yildirim B, Bozbas A, Ozaras R, Demir K, et al. Sexual transmission of HCV between spouses. Am J Gastroenterol. 2005;100:821–4.
5. Terrault NA, Dodge JL, Murphy EL, Tavis JE, Kiss A, Levin TR, Gish RG, Busch MP, Reingold AL, Alter MJ. Sexual transmission of hepatitis C virus among monogamous heterosexual couples: the HCV partners study. Hepatology. 2013;57(3):881–9.
6. Vandelli C, Renzo F, Romano L, Tisminetzky S, De Palma M, Stroffolini T, et al. Lack of evidence of sexual transmission of hepatitis C among monogamous couples: results of a 10-year prospective follow-up study. Am J Gastroenterol. 2004;99:855–9.
7. Filippini P, Coppola N, Scolastico C, et al. Does HIV infection favor the sexual transmission of hepatitis C? Sex Transm Dis. 2001;28:725–9.
8. Briat A, Dulioust E, Galimand J, et al. Hepatitis C virus in the semen of men coinfected with HIV-1: prevalence and origin. AIDS. 2005;19:1827–35.
9. Savasi V, Ferrazzi E, Fiore S. Reproductive assistance for infected couples with bloodborne viruses. Placenta. 2008;29 Suppl B:160–5. Review.
10. Halfon P, Giorgetti C, Bourlière M, et al. Medically assisted procreation and transmission of hepatitis C virus: absence of HCV RNA in purified sperm fraction in HIV co-infected patients. AIDS. 2006;20:241–6.
11. Bourlet T, Lornage J, Maertens A, et al. Prospective evaluation of the threat related to the use of seminal fractions from hepatitis C virus-infected men in assisted reproductive techniques. Hum Reprod. 2009;24:530–5.
12. Decree of May 10. 2001. Prise en charge en assistance médicale à la procréation des patients à risque viral. Page 7735. Arrêté du 10 mai 2001. Journal Officiel de la République Française, 15 mai 2001.
13. Bourlet T, Levy R, Laporte S, et al. Multicenter quality control for the detection of hepatitis C virus RNA in seminal plasma specimens. J Clin Microbiol. 2003;41:789–93.
14. Garrido N, Meseguer M, Remohí J, Simón C, Pellicer A. Semen characteristics in human immunodeficiency virus (HIV)- and hepatitis C (HCV)-seropositive males: predictors of the success of viral removal after sperm washing. Hum Reprod. 2005;20:1028–34.
15. Azzari C, Resti M, Moriondo M, Ferrari R, Lionetti P, Vierucci A. Vertical transmission of HCV is related to maternal peripheral blood mononuclear cell infection. Blood. 2000;96:2045–8.

16. Maggi F, Fornai C, Vatteroni ML, et al. Differences in hepatitis C virus quasispecies composition between liver, peripheral blood mononuclear cells and plasma. J Gen Virol. 1997;78:1521–5.
17. Okuda M, Hino K, Korenaga M, Yamaguchi Y, Katoh Y, Okita K. Differences in hypervariable region 1 quasispecies of hepatitis C virus in human serum, peripheral blood mononuclear cells, and liver. Hepatology. 1999;29:217–22.
18. Roque Afonso AM, Jiang J, Penin F, et al. Nonrandom distribution of hepatitis C virus quasispecies in plasma and peripheral blood mononuclear cell subsets. J Virol. 1999;73:9213–21.
19. Savasi V, Parrilla B, Ratti M, Oneta M, Clerici M, Ferrazzi E. Hepatitis C virus RNA detection in different semen fractions of HCV/HIV-1 co-infected men by nested PCR. Eur J Obstet Gynecol Reprod Biol. 2010;151:52–5.
20. Weigel MM, Gentili M, Beichert M, Friese K, Sonnenberg-Schwan U. Reproductive assistance to HIV-discordant couples—the German approach. Eur J Med Res. 2001;28:259–62.
21. Englert Y, Lesage B, Van Vooren JP, et al. Medically assisted reproduction in the presence of chronic viral diseases. Hum Reprod Update. 2004;10:149–62. Review.
22. ASRM—The Practice Committee of the American Society for Reproductive Medicine. Hepatitis and reproduction. Fertil Steril. 2008;90:S226–35.

Chapter 7
Laboratory Safety During Assisted Reproduction in Patients with a Bloodborne Virus

Asma Sassi, Fabienne Devreker, and Yvon Englert

Risk of Cross-Contamination and Nosocomial Transmission

Worldwide, hepatitis B virus (HBV) accounts for an estimated 370 million chronic infections, hepatitis C virus (HCV) for an estimated 130 million, and HIV for an estimated 40 million. HBV, HCV and HIV share common routes of transmission, even if nonsexual transmission is more common in HCV transmission. The prevalence of potentially infectious individuals varies depending on the virus involved, the geographic region and the population subgroups. In developed countries, the general population prevalence of HBV is <0.5%, HCV 1% and HIV 0.15% [1]. Sub-Saharan Africa accounts for most (65%) HIV infections worldwide and has a high prevalence of chronic HBV infection. The population prevalence of HIV is 20% in Southern Africa and at least 8% of the population in these areas are chronically infected, with 70–90% having serological evidence of previous HBV infection [2]. The highest prevalence of HCV infection has been reported from

A. Sassi, MD • F. Devreker, MD, PhD • Y. Englert, MD, PhD, MBA (✉)
Laboratory for Research in Human Reproduction, Medicine Faculty,
Department of Obstetrics and Gynecology, Hôpital Erasme,
Université Libre de Bruxelles (ULB), Route de Lennik, 808,
Brussels 1070, Belgium
e-mail: Fabienne.Devreker@erasme.ulb.ac.be;
yvon.englert@erasme.ulb.ac.be

© Springer International Publishing Switzerland 2016   157
A. Borini, V. Savasi (eds.), *Assisted Reproductive Technologies and Infectious Diseases*,
DOI 10.1007/978-3-319-30112-9_7

Northern Africa (particularly Egypt), and has been found in 25–30% of HIV-positive persons and 72–95% of injection drug users [2–5]. Some Asian countries have a high incidence of BBV carriers. Heterosexual intercourse represents the major vector of HIV transmission worldwide. The risk of seroconversion after an initial negative screen in co-habiting couples participating in an ART programme is negligible. The incidence in this population of hepatitis B surface antigen was 0.28%, hepatitis C antibody 0.33%, and HIV 0.007% [6].

Viral transmission risk via ART is possible and has been reported. Cross-contamination between infected and uninfected patients and samples can potentially occur during clinical procedures and during subsequent laboratory procedures such as insemination, injection, incubation and cryopreservation [7, 8]. HBV is known to be present in many body compartments including blood, semen and vaginal secretions depending on the viral concentration [7, 9]. In addition, HBV (and HCV) can remain viable in dried blood on environmental surfaces at room temperature [3]. A case has been reported of an acute viral hepatitis B in a woman following artificial insemination with a sperm donor, which was subsequently found to be positive for hepatitis B surface antigen [10]. The infection of women whose embryos were exposed to HBV in contaminated human serum present in the culture medium during in vitro fertilisation (IVF) has also been reported [11]. In vitro and in vivo data suggest that the risk of HBV integration, and subsequent replication and expression, remains during IVF and intracytoplasmic sperm injection (ICSI) procedures as germ cells may be vectors for the vertical transmission of HBV [9, 12, 13]. HBV DNA, HBV RNA and HBsAg were found in oocytes and embryos of couples with at least one HBsAg-seropositive partner [12, 13]. HBV can integrate into human sperm and oocytes. Human sperm-mediated HBV genes are able to replicate and express themselves, as suggested by the detection and expression of the HBV X gene in one- and two-cell embryos from golden hamster oocytes fertilised in vitro with human spermatozoa carrying HBV DNA [14]. The entire HBV genome, introduced via pronuclear DNA microinjection, was integrated into mouse F1 hybrid embryos and stably transmitted to progeny until the F10 generation [15]. HBV DNA sequences are able to pass through the zona pellucida and oolemma to enter mouse oocytes and are also able to integrate into their chromosomes [16].

Performing ART in a patient with HCV infection may also lead to a possible risk of nosocomial contamination. In fact, HCV RNA was detected in unfertilised oocytes and in follicular fluid and culture media from HCV-positive women irrespective of the degree of blood contamination [17, 18]. HCV was also present in the seminal plasma of chronically HCV-infected males at varying prevalence [19] with no correlation with HCV virus load [20]. Two cases of nosocomial transmission of HCV in patients attending the ART centre for ICSI/FIV have been reported. In both cases the contaminated patient had had follicular puncture immediately after the HCV infected patient puncture one [21]. It should be remembered that HCV is an RNA virus and has no reverse transcriptase activity; therefore, it cannot succeed in DNA integration within infected cells, sperm or embryos [22]. One case of an HCV-infected newborn out of 30 born to HCV- and polymerase chain reaction (PCR)-positive women undergoing ICSI cycles has been reported and none of those born to PCR-negative females was infected [23]. HIV virus is present in semen as a free virus in the seminal plasma and as a cell-associated virus in the non-sperm cells. HIV may be able to attach to or infect spermatozoa, although this issue is controversial [7, 24]. HIV infection in artificial insemination with a sperm donor has been reported [25–27]. Transmission of HIV by artificial insemination by donor semen was first described in Australia by Stewart et al. [28], then by Chiasson et al. [25] in the USA. These accidents demonstrated early in the epidemic that sperm alone, independently of any sexual contact, can transmit the virus with very similar frequencies to situations of occasional sexual intercourse.

The blood plasma viral load of HIV is known to be related to the risk of HIV transmission [29, 30]; however, viral loads in semen and in blood plasma may be discordant [31]. The virus can persist in semen even during antiretroviral therapy and with an undetectable blood viral load [29, 32–34]. HIV RNA may be amplified in semen, when undetectable in plasma, in 2–8 % of patients under highly active antiretroviral therapy (HAART) [35, 36]. The female genital tract also represents a distinct compartment for HIV-1 replication/evolution. Genital shedding of the virus was demonstrated in 25 % of women with an undetectable plasma viral load [37]. The presence of HIV-1 in follicular fluids, flushes and cumulus oophorus cells of HIV-1-seropositive women during ART has been reported, which represents a cross-contamination risk within the laboratory setting [24, 38].

BBV Infection Risk Related to Cryopreservation

Although not yet reported, the cryopreservation of gametes and embryos in liquid nitrogen presents a risk of cross-contamination of HIV, HBV and HCV to other samples. In fact, these viruses are well known to have the ability to survive, and retain their virulence, in liquid nitrogen [39]. There have already been reports of the HBV contamination of negative bone marrow samples cryopreserved in the same liquid nitrogen tank as those harvested from an HBV-infected patient. The leakage of the cryopreservation bags used to store the infected bone marrow leads to contamination of the tank and its contents with HBV and with subsequent transmission to patients after transplantation [40, 41]. Cross-contamination may occur during semen processing before freezing in laboratories that use containers of polyvinyl alcohol (PVA) sealing powder for multiple patients or donors. In fact, PVA powder may accumulate microorganisms. Tamping straws from different patients into the same powder could result in cross-contamination [42]. The storage of semen in cryovials placed in direct contact with liquid nitrogen may not be safe, as cryovials are able to absorb up to 1 ml of potentially contaminated liquid nitrogen if their caps cannot maintain their seal [40]. Straws may leak or shatter during freezing or blow open during thawing and those that are inadequately sealed could absorb contaminated nitrogen [14, 42]. The type of straws and the sealing system and instruments used are also important. Letur-Könirsch et al. [39] have evaluated the safety of three types of straws under cryopreservation conditions: polyvinyl chloride (PVC), polyethylene terephthalate glycol (PETG) and high-security ionomeric resin (IR) straws. Only the heat-sealed ionomeric resin straws were found to be safe against leakage of HIV-1 into the surrounding medium [39]. Sealing PVC and PETG straws ultrasonically could incur the risk of not ensuring their impermeability [39, 43].

Safety Measurements

Patient admittance to ART treatment cycles must be regulated by physicians and the laboratory staff must be informed about the risks of handling potentially infected biological material. Certain strategies should be established to ensure the safety of ART and significantly reduce the risk of BBV infection and cross-contamination.

The first step consists of routinely screening patients for human HIV, HBC, HCV and other sexually transmissible diseases before processing or cryopreservation gametes and embryos [7, 44]. Screening is mandatory only for gamete donors, which is not the case for the donation of reproductive cells between partners who have an intimate physical relationship ([45], Annex III). However, systematic screening of couples attending assisted reproduction centres is strongly recommended, as it confers many benefits from the ethical and medico-legal standpoints [7, 8].

Where HIV-1 and -2, hepatitis B or hepatitis C test results are positive or unavailable, or if screening is refused by one or both partners, samples should be processed in a separate laboratory or designed space within the same laboratory, utilising a separate storage tank to minimise the risk of cross-contamination [7, 8, 46]. There is good evidence for recommending the use of antiviral drugs in an HIV-infected partner, to reduce HIV viraemia [47] and to use sperm-washing methods if the male is HIV+ or HCV+. In fact, reduction of HIV and/or HCV shedding in semen by density gradient centrifugation followed by swim-up is an efficient method [31, 32, 48–52] and should be performed to decrease the viral load before using and freezing the semen samples.

The sperm-washing procedure consists of density gradient centrifugation followed by a sperm swim-up step to separate motile sperm from free HIV and HIV-infected somatic cells [53, 54]. Virological testing of the sperm fraction using a PCR technique for the presence of residual detectable HIV before its use for insemination can provide an added measure of safety, as up to 8 % of samples may contain residual virus after the procedure [52]. Very sensitive RT-nested PCR assay for the detection of HIV-1 RNA in different parts of semen for which the sensitivity for HIV-1 RNA detection is 20–50 HIV-1 RNA copies per millilitre have been developed [32]. HIV-1 RNA could be detected even after swim-up and the inhibition of HIV-1 RNA amplification is relatively common; thus, when using PCR techniques for semen validation, inhibition of the reaction must be controlled by using an internal control that is well targeted at exploring the detection limit of the method. Extraction techniques using silica or resine breads seemed to increase the assay performance because of better washing [55]. The sperm-washing procedure could also be used in cases of sperm retrieval where sperm volume and density are low, allowing the treatment with testicular spermatozoa in azoospermic HIV-positive men [56–59]. HCV RNA was detected in 20 % of seminal plasma samples from HCV viraemic patients, but not in any seminal cells or motile spermatozoa fractions [31]. After density gradient centrifugation was either followed or not followed by a swim-up step, no HCV RNA was found in the purified 90 % fraction of the sperm, which is the one used for insemination [31, 60]. Even if no effective vaccine against HCV is available, ribavirin and peginterferon could be used to decrease the viral load before fertility treatment in a PCR-positive, HCV-infected partner (48 weeks). Pregnancy should be deferred for an additional 6 months after the conclusion of therapy, regardless of which partner is undergoing the treatment [46]. In male HBV patients, sperm-washing is not necessary for preventing the risk of sexual transmission unless the female partner has not been effectively vaccinated against HBV and in this case ART should be delayed until vaccination has taken place [7, 9, 46].

If the woman is infected by the HBV, the couple must be warned about the necessity of the specific vaccination of their newborn [44]. A systematic review of the literature has shown that lamivudine use in HBV carrier-mothers with a high degree of infectiousness in late pregnancy effectively prevented HBV intrauterine infection and mother-to-child transmission [61].

Universal precautions and adherence to strict safety guidelines should be applied in all ART laboratories, but those dedicated to chronic carriers of viruses should be equipped with the whole range of adapted facilities for handling of gametes, embryos or ovarian or testicular cells for ART [7, 8]. Preimplantation diagnosis may even be performed if needed [62]. To further minimise the risks of cross-contamination, infected patients should be separately treated in a dedicated facilities or at different time from non infected patients [7, 8, 63–65]. Infected patients can be seen at the end of the programme for vaginal echography, oocyte retrieval, transfer and insemination [7]. Vaginal ultrasound probes should be covered with a protective sheath and wiped with a germicide-impregnated tissue before and after each patient is scanned [66]. A separate adapted laboratory devoted to infected patients, with an airtight chamber and safety access procedures could be set apart for treating the biological material of patients (semen, oocytes and embryos) when HIV, HCV or HBV carriers are involved. A vertical laminar flow cabinet for viral culture with 100 % recirculation of filtered air was adapted with a microscope and video vision to provide the laboratory workers with a safe workplace [7, 8]. The laboratory designs include facilities for cleaning and disinfection; working surfaces and equipment used should be cleaned with additional non-embryotoxic disinfecting agents [7, 8].

Some other general protective measures should be applied, such as the use of laboratory clothing, non-toxic gloves and masks, eye and face protection where appropriate, and the use of cryogloves when handling cryogenic materials. A fume-hood should be used when using fixatives. Mechanical pipetting devices should be used for one procedure only and never for more than one patient at a time. Mouth pipetting should be prohibited. Needles and other sharps should be handled with caution and discarded in special containers. Any non-disposable equipment should be sterilised using non-embryotoxic products. Access to the laboratory should be limited to authorised personnel only [7, 8, 44, 46, 67].

During storage, proper measures should be taken to safeguard against the risk of cross-contamination. A system of separate storage should be considered [7, 8, 17]. Containers used for cryopreservation must be guaranteed by manufacturers to withstand freezing temperatures. Any straws found to be defective after thawing should not be used in ART. Adequate sealing is essential and should be checked carefully before freezing. A procedure whereby straws are heat-sealed at both ends should be implemented. The safety of heat-sealed shatterproof CBSTM ionomeric resin straws for the cryopreservation of semen-containing HCV [68] and HIV-1 RNA [39] have been demonstrated, with no reported cases of cross-contamination. The use of "double bagging" to store cryovials inside a second skin, such as those called Cryoflex, to prevent the direct contact of the cryocontainer with the liquid nitrogen, is recommended [40, 46]. The use of vapour storage for both oocytes and sperm may be a viable alternative to the storage of gametes and/or embryos in liquid nitrogen alone, which has the potential to become contaminated [40, 46, 69–71]. PVA powder sealing should be used for one patient only. Straws should be decontaminated after sealing [43, 68]. Incubators should be frequently cleaned and sterilised. Nitrogen tanks are recommended to be cleaned and sanitised at least every year [67]. The exterior surface of straws should be sterilised before cutting with the use of sterile scissors to open the straws. Only one patient biological sample should be processed for cryopreservation at a time, at a workstation separated from other biological samples. In addition, to diminish the risks further, ART using cryopreserved sperm should involve a semen preparation protocol employing density gradients and sperm-washing techniques [31, 60].

Concern About Natural Conception in HIV-Serodiscordant Couples

For serodiscordant couples with no infertility factors, natural conception could be an alternative to assisted reproduction under certain conditions. If the woman is the infected partner, conception is possible by auto-insemination with no risk to the partner. Some authors are in favour of conception by unprotected sexual intercourse limited to the fertile days for HIV-serodiscordant couples treated by HAART where there is an undetectable viral load [72, 73].

The Swiss HIV Commission stated in its guidelines that: "The risk of sexual transmission of HIV is negligibly low if three conditions are met: (1) the HIV-infected patient is receiving antiretroviral therapy with excellent adherence; (2) blood viral load has consistently been undetectable (<40 copies per ml) for more than 6 months; and (3) no sexually transmitted diseases (STDs) are present in either of the partners" [36].

Gray et al. [74] showed a lack of sexual HIV transmission through unprotected intercourse in couples in which males had viral load values <1500 HIV RNA copies/ml and estimated the average risk of heterosexual HIV transmission to be 0.001–0.0001 per sexual contact [74]. However, it is worth noting that the average number of acts of sexual intercourse necessary to achieve pregnancy at 26–35 years of age for a couple with normal fertility is hence 3–10 and thus for a risk of HIV transmission of 0.0001 per unprotected act of sexual intercourse, the risk of seroconversion would then be 0.001 per pregnancy [75]. This risk could be higher, as fertility could be altered in HIV-positive persons because of the infection itself or the potential impact of the HAART on ovarian function and the sperm quality and so the required numbers of cycles necessary to conceive are higher, especially if the woman is older [75]. Furthermore, to obtain an estimated risk of transmission of 0.001–0.0001 per sexual contact, a series of 3000–30,000 natural pregnancies would be needed to truly establish the safety of such an approach [72]. The couple should be informed that there is much better controlled experience with "sperm-washing" procedures, as natural conception is still registered in small series [72].

Antiretroviral pre-exposure prophylaxis is a promising approach for preventing human immunodeficiency virus type 1 (HIV-1) infection in heterosexual populations. A randomised trial of oral antiretroviral therapy for use as pre-exposure prophylaxis among HIV-1-serodiscordant heterosexual couples from Kenya and Uganda, enrolling 1584 couples randomly assigned to TDF, 1579 to TDF-FTC and 1584 to placebo, and followed monthly for up to 36 months, showed that the once daily intake of tenofovir (TDF) or a combination tenofovir–emtricitabine (TDF–FTC) are respectively associated with a relative reduction of 67 and 75 % in the incidence of HIV-1. The HIV-1-seropositive partners were not receiving antiretroviral therapy and did not meet Kenyan or Ugandan guidelines for initiation of antiretroviral therapy. TDF was given at a dose of 300 mg, and FTC 200 mg [76].

Whetham et al. [77] reported the first UK use of pre-exposure prophylaxis for conception (PrEP-C) in 32 male-positive/female-negative couples. The PrEP-C consists on TDF–FTC intake by the female at protocol-designated times before ± after timed ovulatory intercourse. Eleven pregnancies in ten couples have been obtained with no HIV transmission. Mugo NR et al. [78] showed the safety of PrEP with TDF alone or combination FTC+TDF taken at conception, as differences in pregnancy incidence, birth outcomes, and infant growth were not statistically different when compared with placebo [78].

Guidelines were proposed to further reduce the risk of sexual transmission:

1. The male partner being successfully treated, with undetectable HIV RNA in the plasma (<50 copies/ml) for at least 6 months, without the need for HIV RNA testing in semen
2. No current symptoms of genital infections
3. No unprotected sex with other partners
4. Use of a luteinising hormone (LH) test in the urine to determine the optimal time of conception (36 h after LH peak)
5. PrEP with TDF (300 mg), first dose at LH peak and a second dose 24 h later with intercourse the evening of the second dose

After six unsuccessful attempts a fertility evaluation is suggested [79].

Attitude Regarding Gamete Donors

According to Commission Directive 2006/17/EC [45] Annex III, of 8 February 2006 implementing Directive 2004/23/EC of the European Parliament and of the Council regarding certain technical requirements for the donation, procurement and testing of human tissues and cells, gamete donors other than partners must be screened for sexually transmitted infections and must be negative for HIV-1 and -2, HCV, HBV and syphilis on a serum or plasma sample, tested in accordance with Annex II, point 1.1, and sperm donors must additionally be negative for chlamydia on a urine sample tested by the nucleic acid amplification technique (NAT). Blood samples must be obtained at the time of donation. Sperm donations other than from partners are quarantined for a minimum of 180 days, after which repeat testing is required. No quarantine is needed when blood NAT testing have been performed on the day of donation. Human T-cell lymphotropic virus type I (HTLV-I) antibody testing must be performed for donors living in or originating from high-incidence areas or with sexual partners. Under certain circumstances, additional testing may be required, depending on the donor's travel and exposure history and the characteristics of the tissue or cells donated (e.g. RhD, malaria, cytomegalovirus, *Trypanosoma cruzi*).

According to the guidelines for Gamete and Embryo Donation published by the Practice Committee of the American Society for Reproductive Medicine [80], the quarantining of oocytes is not practical. All potential recipient couples should be offered the option of cryopreserving and quarantining embryos derived from donor oocytes for 180 days, with release of the embryos only after the donor has been retested, with confirmed negative results. However, couples also should be informed that embryo cryopreservation may significantly reduce implantation rates. The recipient couple should be appropriately counselled in the event of seroconversion of the oocyte donor after cryopreservation of the embryos. Attitudes regarding oocyte cryopreservation for donation should be changed regarding the efficiency of NAT testing and the contemporary vitrification methods [81]. Cobo et al. [82] showed that the delivery rate (DR) per warming cycle using vitrified embryos developed from vitrified oocytes or vitrified embryos derived from fresh oocytes are comparable (33.8 % vs 30.9 %) and concluded that vitrification at the early cleavage or blastocyst stage of embryos obtained from previously vitrified oocytes has no effect on the DR/warming cycle. Dominguez et al. [83] also reported that oocyte vitrification does not disturb embryonic metabolomic profiles and that the outcome of cryotransfer of embryos developed from vitrified oocytes (double vitrification) has no impact on delivery rates.

BBV Infection Risk and Attitude Regarding Health Care Workers

The main risk to health care workers (HCWs) is through needle-stick and other percutaneous and mucocutaneous exposures, which are frequent, and under-reported [84]. Laboratory technicians and hospital nurses are the most frequently exposed groups [1, 84, 85]. The average risk of HIV transmission after a percutaneous exposure to HIV-infected blood has been estimated to be approximately 0.3% (95% confidence interval [CI], 0.2–0.5%) and that after mucous membrane exposure it is approximately 0.09% (95% CI, 0.006–0.5%) [4]. Exposure to contaminated needlesticks among healthcare workers has demonstrated that HBV is 100 times more infectious than HIV and HCV is ten times more infectious than HIV [2]. This risk is related to the frequency of contaminated exposures, the prevalence of disease in the source populations, the risk of transmission given exposure to an infected source and the effectiveness of post-exposure management [1].

Post-exposure prophylaxis should be offered to all persons who have sustained a mucosal or parenteral exposure to HIV from a known infected source as urgently as possible and, at most, within 72 h after exposure [86, 87]. Antiretroviral agents from six classes of drugs are currently available to treat HIV infection. These include the nucleoside and nucleotide reverse-transcriptase inhibitors (NRTIs), non-nucleoside reverse-transcriptase inhibitors (NNRTIs), protease inhibitors (PIs), a fusion inhibitor (FI), an integrase strand transfer inhibitor (INSTI) and a chemokine (C-C motif) receptor 5 (CCR5) antagonist [4]. In low-risk exposure, the treatment regimen consists of TDF (300 mg once daily) with FTC (Emtriva; 200 mg once daily); a combination drug available as Truvada (300/200-mg tablet once daily) or zidovudine (Retrovir; 300 mg twice daily) with lamivudine (Epivir; 150 mg twice daily); a combination drug available as Combivir (300/150-mg tablet twice daily) should be started. In high-risk exposure, the treatment regimen consists of TDF (300 mg once daily) with FTC (200 mg once daily) or zidovudine (300 mg twice daily) with lamivudine (150 mg twice daily), plus lopinavir/ritonavir (Kaletra; 400/100 mg, two tablets twice daily) or atazanavir (Reyataz;

400 mg once daily). All these regimens should be started within 72 h after exposure for 4 weeks [86].

In non-vaccinated HCWs or HCWs with an unknown antibody response to vaccination exposed to an HbsAg-positive or an untested source patient, post-exposure prophylaxis consists of a single dose of hepatitis B immune globulin, 0.06 ml per kg intramuscularly within 24 h of exposure, followed by hepatitis B vaccine series [86]. No effective post-exposure prophylaxis is available for HCV, and neither interferon nor immune globulin is recommended; however, it is crucial to identify HCV exposure and infection in health care [1, 85, 86].

The psychological impact of needlesticks or exposure to blood or body fluid should not be underestimated for HCWs [4, 7]. HCWs frequently experience intrusive thoughts, problems concentrating, sleeping difficulties, anger and a decrease in sexual desire. Some can even react aggressively as an expression of fear for their own safety [1, 7, 85]. Although the hepatitis viruses are more easily transmissible, the fear of HIV infection is the major cause of stress and anxiety experienced by many HCWs. Special attention should be given to motivation and training of the fertility clinic staff who are not accustomed to handling infected patients [7]. Vaccination of the medical staff against hepatitis is recommended [44].

Legitimacy of BBV Screening Before Infertility Treatment

Testing patients and gamete donors for HIV and other sexually transmitted diseases is recommended to be routinely adopted before treatment and gamete cryopreservation by the American Society for Reproductive Medicine practice guidelines, ESHRE guidelines for good practice in IVF laboratories 2000, the Commission Directive of the European Parliament and of the Council as regards certain technical requirements for the donation, procurement and testing of human tissues and cells (2004/23/EC and 2006/17/EC, Annex III). According to the latter, this screening must be performed for the donor other than the partner or the partner donor in the non-direct use of gametes, when reproductive cells are to be processed and/or stored and will result in the cryo-preservation of embryos. However, from the ethical and medico-legal standpoints, all couples planning to have a child should be strongly encouraged to be screened for potentially transmittable infections before treatment, as recommended by the American Society for Reproductive Medicine practice guidelines, and many authors [7, 8, 68, 88]. The screening for BBV before ART is man-datory in belgium, however. This practice should be considered good medical practice, as the means of significantly reducing the risk of HIV transmission to an uninfected partner and to offspring are available: vaccination of the uninfected partner and neonates for HBV, decreasing the viral load of HCV in the pregnant female, which is associated with a minor risk of vertical transmission of HCV [23], or simply informing and counselling patients. Measures can be taken to inform these patients of their condition, prognosis and treatment, refer them to an appropriate physician and counsel them about their reproductive options and the safer reproductive choices [7, 89]. This requires the presence of a multidisciplinary team [7, 64, 89].

Multidisciplinary teams are essential in giving a comprehen-sive approach to patients planning a child while chronically ill with a transmissible and potentially lethal disease. The team in Brussels includes an assisted reproduction clinician, a biologist, a specialist in internal medicine, an obstetrician and a paediatrician all specialised in HIV patients, in addition to a psychologist and the head of the Virology Laboratory and the AIDS Reference Laboratory at the Université Libre de Bruxelles. These profession-als are all working within the same academic hospital. All requests and patients' files are reviewed collectively [7, 89]. Healthcare professionals should provide reproductive counselling, taking into consideration the following aspects: the need to minimise the risk of transmission to the uninfected partner and/or offspring; enabling informed reproductive choices; informing couples about the risks of HIV transmission and the chances of pregnancy, with both natural and medically assisted conception; preparing couples for the psychological impact of assisted conception (availability, duration of treatment, failure and logistics); discussing the possi-bility of fostering or adoptive parenting and informing and advis-ing couples about the risks of sexual and vertical transmission of other frequently associated agents, such as hepatitis B or C [72].

Few people refuse these tests if offered in a non-repressive environment (no refusal has been observed in Brussels in 15 years). In the literature, rates of individuals refusing to undergo screening range from 0.5 to 6 %, probably according to the political and social context [1, 46]. Couples should consider BBV testing as part of responsible parenting and non-discriminatory if they know they will be hosted with respect and be correctly counselled and supported to optimise the control of their disease and the security of their uninfected partner and offspring. Moreover, screening enables patients presenting a risk to HCWs and other patients to be identified pre-treatment, thereby minimising the risk of transmission and cross-contamination when blood sampling, operating, laboratory processing and storing gametes and embryos.

Conclusion

Even if universal precautions are practised, a zero risk does not exist [7, 8, 68]. Patients are free to refuse the screening, but in these cases the centre should handle their gametes and embryos as those of patients who are chronic viral carriers [7, 90, 91]. The screening should not result in discrimination; fertility services should not be withheld from these individuals. The individual should always be referred to a centre that has the capacity to provide the necessary resources.

References

1. Moloughney BW. Transmission and postexposure management of bloodborne virus infections in the health care setting: where are we now? CMAJ. 2001;165(4):445–51.
2. Matthews PC, Geretti AM, Goulder PJ, et al. Epidemiology and impact of HIV coinfection with hepatitis B and hepatitis C viruses in Sub-Saharan Africa. J Clin Virol. 2014;61(1):20–33.
3. Alter MJ. Epidemiology of viral hepatitis and HIV co-infection. J Hepatol. 2006;44(1 Suppl):S6–9.

4. Kuhar DT, Henderson DK, Struble KA, et al. Updated US Public Health Service guidelines for the management of occupational exposures to human immunodeficiency virus and recommendations for postexposure prophylaxis. Infect Control Hosp Epidemiol. 2013;34(9):875–92.

5. Mathers BM, Degenhardt L, Phillips B, et al. Global epidemiology of injecting drug use and HIV among people who inject drugs: a systematic review. Lancet. 2008;372(9651):1733–45.

6. Hughes C, Grundy K, Emerson G, et al. Viral screening at the time of each donation in ART patients: is it justified? Hum Reprod. 2011;26(11):3169–72.

7. Englert Y, Lesage B, Van Vooren JP, et al. Medically assisted reproduction in the presence of chronic viral diseases. Hum Reprod Update. 2004;10(2):149–62.

8. Gilling-Smith C, Emiliani S, Almeida P, et al. Laboratory safety during assisted reproduction in patients with blood-borne viruses. Hum Reprod. 2005;20(6):1433–8.

9. Lutgens SP, Nelissen EC, van Loo IH, et al. To do or not to do: IVF and ICSI in chronic hepatitis B virus carriers. Hum Reprod. 2009;24(11):2676–8.

10. Berry WR, Gottesfeld RL, Alter HJ, et al. Transmission of hepatitis B virus by artificial insemination. JAMA. 1987;257(8):1079–81.

11. Quint WG, Fetter WP, van Os HC, et al. Absence of hepatitis B virus (HBV) DNA in children born after exposure of their mothers to HBV during in vitro fertilization. J Clin Microbiol. 1994;32(4):1099–100.

12. Hu XL, Zhou XP, Qian YL, et al. The presence and expression of the hepatitis B virus in human oocytes and embryos. Hum Reprod. 2011;26(7):1860–7.

13. Nie R, Jin L, Zhang H, et al. Presence of hepatitis B virus in oocytes and embryos: a risk of hepatitis B virus transmission during in vitro fertilization. Fertil Steril. 2011;95(5):1667–71.

14. Ali BA, Huang TH, Xie QD. Detection and expression of hepatitis B virus X gene in one and two-cell embryos from golden hamster oocytes in vitro fertilized with human spermatozoa carrying HBV DNA. Mol Reprod Dev. 2005;70(1):30–6.

15. Bagis H, Arat S, Mercan HO, et al. Stable transmission and expression of the hepatitis B virus total genome in hybrid transgenic mice until F10 generation. J Exp Zool A Comp Exp Biol. 2006;305(5):420–7.

16. Huang TH, Zhang QJ, Xie QD, et al. Presence and integration of HBV DNA in mouse oocytes. World J Gastroenterol. 2005; 11(19):2869–73.

17. Devaux A, Soula V, Sifer C, et al. Hepatitis C virus detection in follicular fluid and culture media from HCV+ women, and viral risk during IVF procedures. Hum Reprod. 2003;18(11):2342–9.

18. Papaxanthos-Roche A, Trimoulet P, Commenges-Ducos M, et al. PCR-detected hepatitis C virus RNA associated with human zona-intact oocytes collected from infected women for ART. Hum Reprod. 2004;19(5):1170–5.

19. Abou-Setta AM. Transmission risk of hepatitis C virus via semen during assisted reproduction: how real is it? Hum Reprod. 2004;19(12):2711–7.

20. Pasquier C, Bujan L, Daudin M, et al. Intermittent detection of hepatitis C virus (HCV) in semen from men with human immunodeficiency virus type 1 (HIV-1) and HCV. J Med Virol. 2003;69(3):344–9.

21. Lesourd F, Izopet J, Mervan C, et al. Transmissions of hepatitis C virus during the ancillary procedures for assisted conception. Hum Reprod. 2000;15(5):1083–5.

22. Steyaert SR, Leroux-Roels GG, Dhont M. Infections in IVF: review and guidelines. Hum Reprod Update. 2000;6(5):432–41.

23. Nesrine F, Saleh H. Hepatitis C virus (HCV) status in newborns born to HCV positive women performing intracytoplasmic sperm injection. Afr Health Sci. 2012;12(1):58–62.

24. Baccetti B, Benedetto A, Collodel G, et al. The debate on the presence of HIV-1 in human gametes. J Reprod Immunol. 1998;41(1–2):41–67.

25. Chiasson MA, Stoneburner RL, Joseph SC. Human immunodeficiency virus transmission through artificial insemination. J Acquir Immune Defic Syndr. 1990;3(1):69–72.

26. Matz B, Kupfer B, Ko Y, et al. HIV-1 infection by artificial insemination. Lancet. 1998;351(9104):728.

27. Wortley PM, Hammett TA, Fleming PL. Donor insemination and human immunodeficiency virus transmission. Obstet Gynecol. 1998;91(4):515–8.

28. Stewart GJ, Tyler JP, Cunningham AL, et al. Transmission of human T-cell lymphotropic virus type III (HTLV-III) by artificial insemination by donor. Lancet. 1985;2(8455):581–5.

29. Coombs RW, Speck CE, Hughes JP, et al. Association between culturable human immunodeficiency virus type 1 (HIV-1) in semen and HIV-1 RNA levels in semen and blood: evidence for compartmentalization of HIV-1 between semen and blood. J Infect Dis. 1998;177(2):320–30.

30. Quinn TC, Wawer MJ, Sewankambo N, Serwadda D, Li C, Wabwire-Mangen F, et al. Viral load and heterosexual transmission of human immunodeficiency virus type 1. Rakai Project Study Group. N Engl J Med. 2000;342:921–9.
31. Pasquier C, Daudin M, Righi L, et al. Sperm washing and virus nucleic acid detection to reduce HIV and hepatitis C virus transmission in serodiscordant couples wishing to have children. AIDS. 2000;14(14):2093–9.
32. Lesage B, Vannin AS, Emiliani S, et al. Development and evaluation of a qualitative reverse-transcriptase nested polymerase chain reaction protocol for same-day viral validation of human immunodeficiency virus type 1 ribonucleic acid in processed semen. Fertil Steril. 2006;86(1):121–8.
33. Le Tortorec A, Dejucq-Rainsford N. [Infection of semen-producing organs by HIV and role in virus dissemination]. Med Sci (Paris). 2010;26(10):861–8.
34. Semprini AE, Vucetich A, Hollander L. Sperm washing, use of HAART and role of elective Caesarean section. Curr Opin Obstet Gynecol. 2004;16(6):465–70.
35. Bujan L, Daudin M, Matsuda T, et al. Factors of intermittent HIV-1 excretion in semen and efficiency of sperm processing in obtaining spermatozoa without HIV-1 genomes. AIDS. 2004;18:757–66.
36. Vernazza PL, Troiani L, Flepp MJ, et al. Potent antiretroviral treatment of HIV-infection results in suppression of the seminal shedding of HIV. The Swiss HIV Cohort Study. AIDS. 2000;14:117–21.
37. Fiore JR, Suligoi B, Saracino A, et al. Correlates of HIV-1 shedding in cervicovaginal secretions and effects of antiretroviral therapies. AIDS. 2003;17(15):2169–76.
38. Bertrand E, Zissis G, Marissens D, et al. Presence of HIV-1 in follicular fluids, flushes and cumulus oophorus cells of HIV-1-seropositive women during assisted-reproduction technology. AIDS. 2004;18(5):823–5.
39. Letur-Könirsch H, Collin G, Sifer C, et al. Safety of cryopreservation straws for human gametes or embryos: a study with human immunodeficiency virus-1 under cryopreservation conditions. Hum Reprod. 2003;18(1):140–4.
40. Clarke GN. Sperm cryopreservation: is there a significant risk of cross-contamination? Hum Reprod. 1999;14(12):2941–3.
41. Tedder RS, Zuckerman MA, Goldstone AH, et al. Hepatitis B transmission from contaminated cryopreservation tank. Lancet. 1995;346(8968):137–40.

42. Russell PH, Lyaruu VH, Millar JD, et al. The potential transmission of infectious agents by semen packaging during storage for artificial insemination. Anim Reprod Sci. 1997;47(4):337–42.
43. Letur-Könirsch H, Collin G, Devaux A, et al. Conservation of human embryos in straws: safety in terms of human immunodeficiency virus. Gynecol Obstet Fertil. 2004;32(4):302–7.
44. Gianaroli L, Plachot M, van Kooij R, et al. ESHRE guidelines for good practice in IVF laboratories. Committee of the Special Interest Group on Embryology of the European Society of Human Reproduction and Embryology. Hum Reprod. 2000;15(10):2241–6.
45. Commission Directive 2006/17/EC of 8 February 2006 implementing Directive 2004/23/EC of the European Parliament and of the Council as regards certain technical requirements for the donation, procurement and testing of human tissues and cells. Official Journal of the European Union, 9.2.2006, L 38/40.
46. Practice Committee of American Society for Reproductive Medicine. Recommendations for reducing the risk of viral transmission during fertility treatment with the use of autologous gametes: a committee opinion. Fertil Steril. 2013;99(2):340–6.
47. Cohen MS, Smith MK, Muessig KE, et al. Antiretroviral treatment of HIV-1 prevents transmission of HIV-1: where do we go from here? Lancet. 2013;382(9903):1515–24.
48. Canto CL, Segurado AC, Pannuti C, et al. Detection of HIV and HCV RNA in semen from Brazilian coinfected men using multiplex PCR before and after semen washing. Rev Inst Med Trop Sao Paulo. 2006;48(4):201–6.
49. Halfon P, Giorgetti C, Bourlière M, et al. Medically assisted procreation and transmission of hepatitis C virus: absence of HCV RNA in purified sperm fraction in HIV co-infected patients. AIDS. 2006;20(2):241–6.
50. Savasi V, Ferrazzi E, Fiore S. Reproductive assistance for infected couples with bloodborne viruses. Placenta. 2008; 29 Suppl B:160–5.
51. Semprini AE, Vucetich A, Persico T. Hepatitis C detection. Lancet. 2001;357(9255):557.
52. Vitorino RL, Grinsztejn BG, de Andrade CA, et al. Systematic review of the effectiveness and safety of assisted reproduction techniques in couples serodiscordant for human immunodeficiency virus where the man is positive. Fertil Steril. 2011;95(5):1684–90.
53. Politch JA, Xu C, Tucker L, Anderson DJ. Separation of human immunodeficiency virus type 1 from motile sperm by the double tube gradient method versus other methods. Fertil Steril. 2004; 81(2):440–7.

54. Semprini AE, Levi-Setti P, Bozzo M, et al. Insemination of HIV-negative women with processed semen of HIV-positive partners. Lancet. 1992;340(8831):1317–9.

55. Pasquier C, Anderson D, Andreutti-Zaugg C, et al. Multicenter quality control of the detection of HIV-1 genome in semen before medically assisted procreation. J Med Virol. 2006;78(7):877–82.

56. Bostan A, Vannin AS, Emiliani S, et al. Development and evaluation of single sperm washing for risk reduction in artificial reproductive technology (ART) for extreme oligospermic HIV positive patients. Curr HIV Res. 2008;6(5):461–5.

57. Bujan L, Daudin M, Moinard N, et al. Azoospermic HIV-1 infected patients wishing to have children: proposed strategy to reduce HIV-1 transmission risk during sperm retrieval and intracytoplasmic sperm injection: Case Report. Hum Reprod. 2007;22(9):2377–81.

58. Nicopoullos JD, Frodsham LC, Ramsay JW, et al. Synchronous sperm retrieval and sperm washing in an intracytoplasmic sperm injection cycle in an azoospermic man who was positive for human immunodeficiency virus. Fertil Steril. 2004;81(3):670–4.

59. Leruez-Ville M, Thiounn N, Poirot C, et al. Intracytoplasmic sperm injection with microsurgically retrieved spermatozoa in azoospermic men infected with human immunodeficiency virus 1 or hepatitis C virus: the EP43 AZONECO ANRS study. Fertil Steril. 2013;99(3):713–7.

60. Levy R, Tardy JC, Bourlet T, et al. Transmission risk of hepatitis C virus in assisted reproductive techniques. Hum Reprod. 2000;15(4):810–6.

61. Shi Z, Yang Y, Ma L, et al. Lamivudine in late pregnancy to interrupt in utero transmission of hepatitis B virus: a systematic review and meta-analysis. Obstet Gynecol. 2010;116(1):147–59.

62. Gonzales-Merino E, Zengbe V, Vannin AS, et al. Preimplantation genetic diagnosis in an HIV-serodiscordant couple carrier for sickle cell disease: lessons from a case report. Clin Genet. 2009;75: 277–81.

63. Ohl J, Partisani M, Wittemer C, et al. Assisted reproduction techniques for HIV serodiscordant couples: 18 months of experience. Hum Reprod. 2003;18(6):1244–9.

64. Shenfield F, Pennings G, Cohen J, et al. Taskforce 8: ethics of medically assisted fertility treatment for HIV positive men and women. Hum Reprod. 2004;19(11):2454–6.

65. Sifer C, Cassuto G, Poncelet C, et al. Risks in medically-assisted procreation in case of positivity for HIV, hepatitis C virus or hepatitis B virus. The French law at the end of 2001. Gynecol Obstet Fertil. 2003;31(5):410–21.

66. Milki AA, Fisch JD. Vaginal ultrasound probe cover leakage: implications for patient care. Fertil Steril. 1998;69(3):409–11.
67. Magli MC, Van den Abbeel E, Lundin K, et al. Revised guidelines for good practice in IVF laboratories. Hum Reprod. 2008;23(6): 1253–62.
68. Maertens A, Bourlet T, Plotton N, et al. Validation of safety procedures for the cryopreservation of semen contaminated with hepatitis C virus in assisted reproductive technology. Hum Reprod. 2004;19(7):1554–7.
69. Amesse LS, Srivastava G, Uddin D, et al. Comparison of cryopreserved sperm in vaporous and liquid nitrogen. J Reprod Med. 2003;48(5):319–24.
70. Cobo A, Romero JL, Pérez S, et al. Storage of human oocytes in the vapor phase of nitrogen. Fertil Steril. 2010;94(5):1903–7.
71. Lim JJ, Shin TE, Song SH, et al. Effect of liquid nitrogen vapor storage on the motility, viability, morphology, deoxyribonucleic acid integrity, and mitochondrial potential of frozen-thawed human spermatozoa. Fertil Steril. 2010;94(7):2736–41.
72. Barreiro P, Castilla JA, Labarga P, Soriano V. Is natural conception a valid option for HIV-serodiscordant couples? Hum Reprod. 2007;22:2353–8.
73. Wilson DP, Law MG, Grulich AE, et al. Relation between HIV viral load and infectiousness: a model-based analysis. Lancet. 2008;372:314–20.
74. Gray RH, Wawer MJ, Brookmeyer R, et al. Probability of HIV-1 transmission per coital act in monogamous, heterosexual, HIV-1-discordant couples in Rakai, Uganda. Lancet. 2001;357:1149–53.
75. Vandermaelen A, Englert Y. Human immunodeficiency virus serodiscordant couples on highly active antiretroviral therapies with undetectable viral load: conception by unprotected sexual intercourse or by assisted reproduction techniques? Hum Reprod. 2010;25(2): 374–9.
76. Baeten JM, Donnell D, Ndase P, et al. Antiretroviral prophylaxis for HIV prevention in heterosexual men and women. N Engl J Med. 2012;367(5):399–410.
77. Whetham J, Taylor S, Charlwood L, et al. Pre-exposure prophylaxis for conception (PrEP-C) as a risk reduction strategy in HIV-positive men and HIV-negative women in the UK. AIDS Care. 2014;26(3):332–6.
78. Mugo NR, Hong T, Celum C, et al. Pregnancy incidence and outcomes among women receiving preexposure prophylaxis for HIV prevention: a randomized clinical trial. JAMA. 2014;312(4):362–71.

79. Savasi V, Mandia L, Laoreti A, et al. Reproductive assistance in HIV serodiscordant couples. Hum Reprod Update. 2013;19(2):136–50.
80. Practice Committee of the American Society for Reproductive Medicine, Practice Committee of the Society for Assisted Reproductive Technology. 2006 guidelines for gamete and embryo donation. Fertil Steril. 2006;86(5 Suppl 1):S38–50.
81. Cobo A. Oocyte vitrification: a watershed in ART. Fertil Steril. 2012;98(3):600–1.
82. Cobo A, Castelló D, Vallejo B, et al. Outcome of cryotransfer of embryos developed from vitrified oocytes: double vitrification has no impact on delivery rates. Fertil Steril. 2013;99(6):1623–30.
83. Dominguez F, Castello D, Remohí J, et al. Effect of vitrification on human oocytes: a metabolic profiling study. Fertil Steril. 2013;99(2):565–72.
84. Eskandarani HA, Kehrer M, Christensen PB. No transmission of blood-borne viruses among hospital staff despite frequent blood exposure. Dan Med J. 2014;61(9):A4907.
85. Deuffic-Burban S, Delarocque-Astagneau E, Abiteboul D, et al. Blood-borne viruses in health care workers: prevention and management. J Clin Virol. 2011;52(1):4–10.
86. Bader MS, McKinsey DS. Postexposure prophylaxis for common infectious diseases. Am Fam Physician. 2013;88(1):25–32.
87. Marrazzo JM, del Rio C, Holtgrave DR, et al. HIV prevention in clinical care settings: 2014 recommendations of the International Antiviral Society-USA Panel. JAMA. 2014;312(4):390–409.
88. Gilling-Smith C, Smith JR, Semprini AE. HIV and infertility: time to treat. There's no justification for denying treatment to parents who are HIV positive. BMJ. 2001;322(7286):566–7.
89. Englert Y, Van Vooren JP, Place I, et al. ART in HIV-infected couples: has the time come for a change of attitude? Hum Reprod. 2001;16(7):1309–15.
90. Ethics Committee of the American Society for Reproductive Medicine. American Society for Reproductive Medicine. Fertil Steril. 2002;77(2).
91. Ethics Committee of the American Society for Reproductive Medicine. Human immunodeficiency virus and infertility treatment. Fertil Steril. 2010;94(1):11–5.

Chapter 8
Accessibility to Reproductive Assistance in Low-Income Countries

Irene Cetin and Arianna Laoreti

Introduction

In the past few years, the global health community has made a great effort to improve maternal and child health in low-income countries, in particular focusing on reproductive health. Although infertility is a critical component of reproductive health, it has often been neglected in these efforts [1].

Worldwide, between 8 and 12 % of the couples suffer from infertility. Contrary to popular belief, primary and secondary infertility are a major health problem in developing countries too, both quantitatively and qualitatively, affecting a high proportion of couples [2].

I. Cetin, MD (✉) • A. Laoreti, MD
Unit of Obstetrics and Gynecology, Department of Mother and Child,
Luigi Sacco, Via G.B. Grassi, 74, Milan 20157, Italy
e-mail: irene.cetin@unimi.it; arianna.laoreti@unimi.it

© Springer International Publishing Switzerland 2016   179
A. Borini, V. Savasi (eds.), *Assisted Reproductive
Technologies and Infectious Diseases*,
DOI 10.1007/978-3-319-30112-9_8

Prevalence of Infertility in Low-Income Countries

Assessing the prevalence, distribution and trends of infertility is an important first step towards shaping evidence-based interventions and policies to reduce the burden of this neglected condition. However, differences in the definition of infertility account for dissimilar estimates of infertility worldwide, both in developed and developing countries.

A recent study analysed household survey data from 277 demographic and reproductive health surveys to reveal global patterns and trends in infertility [3]. The authors used a demographic infertility measure with live birth as the outcome and a 5-year exposure period based on union status, contraceptive use, and desire for a child. As the main results, they found that in 2010 an estimated 48.5 million couples worldwide were infertile. Among women 20–44 years of age who were exposed to the risk of pregnancy, 1.9 % were unable to obtain a live birth (primary infertility). Out of women who had had at least one live birth and were exposed to the risk of pregnancy, 10.5 % were unable to have another child (secondary infertility; Figs. 8.1 and 8.2). Infertility prevalence was highest in South Asia, sub-Saharan Africa, North Africa/Middle East, Central/Eastern Europe and Central Asia. Levels of infertility in 2010 were similar to those in 1990 in most world regions, apart

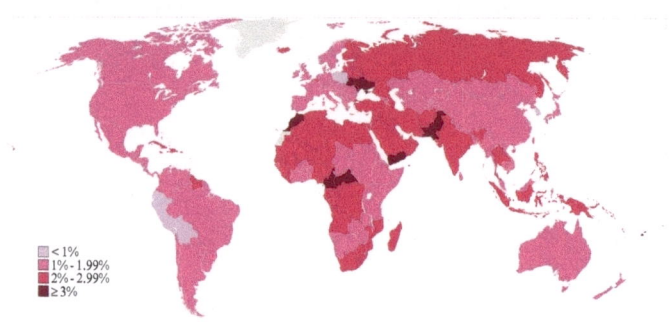

Fig. 8.1 Prevalence of primary infertility among women who seek a child, in 2010. Infertility prevalence relates the female partner; the age-standardised prevalence among women aged 20–44 years [3]

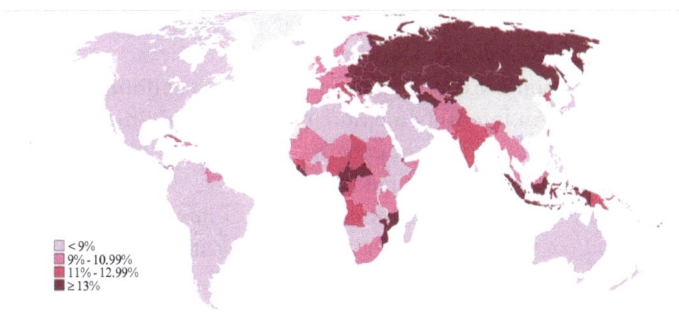

Fig. 8.2 Prevalence of secondary infertility among women who have had a live birth and seek another, in 2010. Infertility prevalence relates to the female partner; the age-standardised prevalence among women aged 20–44 years [3]

from decreases in primary and secondary infertility in sub-Saharan Africa (from 2.7 % in 1900 to 1.9 % in 2010 for primary infertility; from 13.5 to 11.6 % for secondary infertility) and primary infertility in South Asia. Owing to population growth, however, the absolute number of couples affected by infertility increased from 42.0 million in 1990 to 48.5 million in 2010.

The authors of the study reported that their estimate of the global number of couples affected by infertility was lower than that of previous reports. This result is likely because of different definitions of infertility.

Boivin et al. [4] estimated that 72.4 million women were infertile in 2006. They used the median prevalence reported by seven published infertility studies that used a 12- or 24-month definition of infertility. The 12-month prevalence rate of infertility ranged from 6.9 to 9.3 % in less developed countries. Substantial geographical differences in the prevalence were noted, and these differences were largely explained by different environmental, cultural and socioeconomic influences [4].

A previous report by Rutstein and Shah [5] stated that 186 million ever-married women in developing countries (excluding China) were infertile in 2002. This larger number may also be a result of differences in definitions: they included women who may not have been exposed to the risk of pregnancy and women aged 15–20 years and 45–49 years, age groups that have a higher prevalence of infertility than women aged 20–44 years.

In conclusion, we can see the importance of a uniform definition of infertility. An infertility measure based on the ability to become pregnant may have different patterns, trends and levels from those based on the ability to obtain a live birth.

Irrespective of the different definitions of infertility used, there is a broad consensus that prevalence rates for infertility are higher in low-income countries than in developed countries, with the majority of people affected by infertility worldwide living in developing countries and having no access to infertility treatments, which are either unavailable or very costly.

Aetiology and Risk Factors for Infertility in Low-Income Countries

Infertility can be schematically determined by two broad groups of causes. The first group includes genetic, anatomical, hormonal and immunological problems. This group represents the "core" causes of infertility and it is responsible for about 5 % of the prevalence of infertility, with rates similar throughout the world. The second group includes causes that are preventable and their rates therefore differ widely around the world. These preventable causes are largely infection-related and iatrogenic [6].

In a large study performed by the WHO Task Force on the Diagnosis and Treatment of Infertility, 8504 infertile couples in 33 different countries were examined through a standard approach in all participating centres [7, 8]. The authors estimated that in Africa, over 85 % of women had an infertility diagnosis attributable to an infection, compared with 33 % of women worldwide [7]. The type and mode of infection varies from country to country depending on social factors, the health infrastructure, healthcare practices and environmental factors. Also, iatrogenic causes of infertility have higher rates in developing countries, representing approximately 15.5 % of all causes in Africa, compared with 5 % in Western Europe [9].

Most preventable infertility in couples results from one of the factors described in the following paragraphs.

Reproductive Tract Infections

Sexually transmitted diseases (STDs) are prominent risk factors for infertility in developing countries. It has been estimated that approximately 70 % of pelvic infections are caused by STDs, whereas the other 30 % are attributable to pregnancy-related sepsis [10].

A study of 5800 couples in 33 World Health Organisation (WHO) centres in 25 countries showed that almost 50 % of the African couples and 11–15 % of patients in other parts of the world had infectious tubal disease [11].

Studies from Nigeria, South Africa and Egypt have reported prevalence of tubal factor infertility ranging from 42 to 77 % [12].

Similarly, most cases of male factor infertility are caused by previous infections of the male genitourinary tract, and studies conducted in Nigeria have shown a prevalence of male infertility in 26–43 % of cases [13, 14].

The organisms most commonly involved in STD are *Chlamydia trachomatis* and *Neisseria gonorrhoeae* [12, 15]. Moreover, another sexually transmitted organism associated with infertility is HIV-1. Several studies have documented reduced fecundity in HIV-infected individuals [16]. Mechanisms involved include, essentially, tubal factor infertility through the greater susceptibility to other STDs and altered spermatogenesis [17]. Little is known about the possible direct role of HIV virus or antiretroviral therapy in female fertility, especially the negative influence on oocyte quality [16]. In addition, marital instability and polygamy secondary to infertility may in turn increase the spread of HIV-1 infection [18].

Infectious diseases other than STDs may also cause infertility. Among these, tuberculosis is another major cause in both men and women [19] and a high prevalence of pelvic tuberculosis has been reported in studies from the Indian subcontinent [20], leading to tubal pathological conditions.

Genital tuberculosis appears to be an important and common cause of Asherman's syndrome in India, causing oligomenorrhoea or amenorrhoea with infertility. In a study of women with infertility and amenorrhoea/oligomenorrhoea, 68 % had a past history of tuberculosis [21], whereas the prevalence of genital tuberculosis in tubal factor infertility was 49 % in women requesting assisted reproduction [22].

Other infections associated with infertility in developing countries include lepromatous leprosy (which has been associated with an increased risk of semen abnormalities and azoospermia), schistosomiasis and malaria, through a pathogenic mechanism that is still to be explained [6].

Unsafe Abortion and Healthcare Practices

Unsafe abortion is one of the biggest public health issues faced by women worldwide [23]. The WHO defines unsafe abortion as a procedure for terminating a pregnancy performed by persons lacking the necessary skills or in an environment not in conformity with minimal medical standards, or both [24].

Nearly half of all abortions worldwide are unsafe, and nearly all unsafe abortions occur in developing countries (98%). An estimated 21.6 million unsafe abortions took place worldwide in 2008, almost all being performed in developing countries (21.4 millions). In 2008, more than 97% of abortions in Africa and 95% of abortions in Latin America were unsafe [25].

Unsafe abortion can have severe consequences: 20–50% of women have immediate complications (e.g. haemorrhage, sepsis or trauma) and 20–30% suffer upper genital tract infection and become infertile. Unsafe abortions contribute to about 2% of all causes of infertility [21]. Deaths due to unsafe abortion remain close to 13% of all maternal deaths [25].

Unhygienic obstetric practices (other than unsafe abortion) in developing countries are also major contributors to infertility. In sub-Saharan Africa, only 40% of births are attended by trained birth personnel, with severe complications such as trauma and sepsis, both of which increase the risk of future infertility [26].

Sociocultural Factors

The WHO estimates that between 100 and 140 million girls and women worldwide have been subjected to one of the first three types of female genital mutilation [27]. Estimates based on the most recent prevalence data indicate that 91.5 million girls and women above the age of 9 years in Africa are currently living with the consequences of female genital mutilation [28]. There are an estimated three million girls in Africa at risk of undergoing female genital mutilation every year [29].

Female genital mutilation is recognised internationally as a violation of the human rights of girls and women. The practice is mostly carried out by traditional circumcisers, who often play other central roles in communities, such as attending childbirths, and who often have limited knowledge about the principles of aseptic techniques and the underlying anatomy.

The procedure is associated with immediate and long-term complications, which include haemorrhage, urination problems, sepsis, haematocolpos, dysmenorrhoea, dyspareunia, obstructed labour, increased risk of newborn death, fistula formation and infertility [30].

Cultural beliefs such as early marriage, polygamy, aversion to female education and to condoms further contribute indirectly to infertility. There is also a disparity between rural and urban areas with regard to the number of healthcare facilities and access to health care [31].

Nutritional and Environmental Factors

Malnutrition, including micronutrient deficiencies, remains one of the major public health challenges, particularly in developing countries [32]. In 2011, almost 6.9 million children under 5 years of age died worldwide.

Micronutrient deficiencies have been associated with significantly high reproductive risks, ranging from infertility to fetal structural defects and long-term diseases [33].

The WHO estimates that in spite of recent efforts in the prevention and control of micronutrient deficiencies, over two billion people are at risk of vitamin A, iodine and/or iron deficiency globally [34]. Other micronutrient deficiencies of public health concern include zinc, folate and the B vitamins, elements of critical importance for women of reproductive age. In addition, in low-income country settings it is often the case that more than one micronutrient deficiency coexist [32], suggesting the need for simple approaches to correct multiple micronutrient malnutrition (MMN), to decrease malnutrition-related infertility rates.

Environmental factors also have a great impact on fertility and reproductive health, causing about 25 % of deaths and diseases globally, reaching nearly 35 % in regions such as sub-Saharan Africa [35]. A significant proportion of that overall environmental disease burden can be attributed to relatively few key areas of risk. These include: poor water quality and sanitation; vector-borne diseases; poor ambient and indoor air quality; and toxic substances [36].

Psychosocial, Religious and Political Aspects of Infertility

Infertility has a profound effect on women and men worldwide. The psychosocial consequences of infertility for couples in high-income countries have been widely described and include increased symptoms of anxiety and depression, loss of self-esteem, relationship difficulties, diminished sexual satisfaction, reduced life satisfaction and social isolation [37, 38].

In developing countries, those in Africa in particular, communities place a high value on fertility and children. This is the main means of developing the web of relations that is formed with the nuclear and extended family, including the dead and the unborn, the village and the nation. Without children, this web is curtailed and infertile women are considered to be almost non-existent as individuals [39]. Therefore, the inability to conceive represents a devastating burden to the social, economic and personal well-being of those affected, a burden that is disproportionately suffered by the women [40–42]. Womanhood is often defined through motherhood and childless women are frequently stigmatised, leading to a wide range of psycho-social consequences: loss of social status and security, isolation, neglect, domestic violence and abuse, marital instability, problems with gender instability, loss of continuity of family lines, general emotional distress and even suicide [43–49]. Furthermore, as many families in low-income countries depend on children for economic survival, childlessness and having fewer children than the number identified as appropriate are social and public health matters, not just medical problems [50].

Although always negative, the impact of infertility in developing countries varies among different regions and is influenced, among others, by religious, sociocultural and legal factors [12].

Three major religions, Islam, Judaism and Christianity, continue to influence behaviour, attitudes and policy-making. Judaism allows the practice of all techniques of assisted reproduction when the oocyte and spermatozoa originate from the wife and the husband respectively. The attitude towards the practice of assisted reproduction varies among Christian groups, especially those situated in Western Europe and the Americas. Although assisted reproduction is not accepted by the Vatican, it may be practised by Protestant, Anglican and other denominations. According to traditional Christian views, beginning at conception, the embryo has a moral status as a human being, and thus most assisted reproductive technologies (ARTs) are forbidden. Islam dominates the Middle East and North Africa. According to Islam, the procedures of in vitro fertilisation and embryo transfer are acceptable, although they can be performed only within marriage [51].

The rest of Africa and Asia consists of a patchwork of religions, including Buddhism, Hinduism, Taoism and Confucianism. People with Confucian or Buddhist beliefs consider infertility to be retribution for wrongdoing by the man, the woman or even the ancestors [52, 53].

The pattern of religion is changing rapidly in many countries worldwide, as a result of various influences, including migration, disaffection with religion in some populations, and conversion to old or new religions. These changes may lead the physician in the field of reproduction to encounter families with very different beliefs to those that dominated within a given society in the past.

Political context may also have a profound impact on infertility in developing countries. Despite representing a significant problem, there has been no political determination to directly address the problems associated with infertility in these countries. Attention has focused almost exclusively on the extremely high maternal mortality and overpopulation [54].

The overpopulation argument against infertility treatment in developing countries contends that there is already a problem of population growth in the world. From that perspective, infertility treatment not only has negative effects on population growth worldwide, but also diverts limited resources and funds from more important primary health needs [54, 55]. In this context, some believe that the infertile couple should be encouraged to courageously accept their condition of childlessness rather than be offered intervention [56]. Nevertheless, the effect of infertility on an individual's quality of life is huge and it disproportionately affects women and the poor [57]. India has recognised that infertility treatment should not be given a lower priority than other medical conditions and now includes infertility in a comprehensive reproductive and child health programme [58].

It has been argued that, instead of ignoring the problem of infertility in terms of the population growth argument, a better strategy would be to increase the efforts at family planning, with the aim of substantially decreasing fertility rates. At the same time, subfertility needs to be taken seriously and cost-effective techniques of diagnosis and treatment should be implemented.

Prevention of Infertility

Although attitudes among people in high-income countries towards the provision of infertility care in low-income countries have been either uncaring or indifferent, with an emphasis on controlling overpopulation and dealing with limited funding, members of the medical and scientific community increasingly call for action to reduce the global burden of infertility [59–62].

Most authors share the opinion that the first priority should always be prevention rather than cure [60]. Preventive strategies, especially the prevention of pelvic infections caused by STDs or unsafe abortions, which play a major role in the aetiology of infertility, should be regarded as the most important, successful and cost effective strategies for decreasing infertility rates, in addition to strategies to improve women's health in general.

Also, improving education about sexual and reproductive health in adolescents appears to be paramount in reducing the prevalence of infertility. It has been documented that reproductive and sexual events during the teenage years determine the future prospects of fertility [12]. Paradoxically, education not only helps to safeguard future fertility, but also reduces total fertility rates, as studies have shown that education, especially of women, is an important variable determining the desired number of children [63].

Provision of Reproductive Assistance

In 1948, the Universal Declaration of Human Rights stated that "Men and women of full age, without any limitation due to race, nationality or religion, have the right to marry and to raise a family" [64].

Almost 50 years later, at the United Nations International Conference on Population and Development in Cairo, the following statement was made "Reproductive health therefore implies that people have the capability to reproduce and the freedom to decide if, when and how often to do so ... and to have the information and the means to do so..." [65].

In 2004, the World Health Assembly adopted the five core points of the WHO sexual and reproductive health package. One of these was the global need to provide high-quality services for family planning, including infertility services [66]. Furthermore, a stated target to "Achieve by 2015, universal access to reproductive health" represents Goal 5 among the United Nation's Millennium Development Goals (www.un.org) [67].

Despite political and institutional statements, little progress has been made throughout the years towards the attainment of these goals with regard to infertility in developing countries. The reasons are multiple and include the lack of collaboration among non-governmental organisations, civil society groups, the government and the research community; budgetary constraints; and a lack of real political commitment [68].

Two important initiatives highlighted the implications of child-lessness in developing countries and convinced many infertility specialists of the need for accessible infertility care.

In 2001, a meeting was organised the WHO "Medical, Ethical and Social Aspects of Assisted Reproduction" [69]. Among many different recommendations, it was stated that infertility should be recognised as a public health issue worldwide, including in developing countries. Moreover, infertility management should be integrated into national reproductive health education programmes and services and ART should be complementary to other ethically acceptable, social and cultural solutions to infertility.

A second milestone was the foundation of a Special Task Force on "Developing Countries and Infertility" by the European Society of Human Reproduction and Embryology in 2006 [70]. The following objectives were set out:

- To raise awareness surrounding the problem of childlessness in resource-poor countries within the donor community, politicians, funding agencies and research organisations through lobbying and publishing and the general population through information, education and counselling on infertility and its consequences.
- To study the ethical, sociocultural and economic aspects of childlessness and infertility care in resource-poor countries.
- To make infertility diagnosis and infertility treatment, including ARTs, available and accessible to a much larger proportion of the population, by simplifying the diagnostic procedures and simplifying and modifying the ovarian stimulation protocols and in vitro fertilisation procedures.
- To work together with other organisations and societies working in the field of reproductive health to reach the goal of "global access to infertility care".

In 2010, The Walking Egg (www.thewalkingegg.com) was established, a not-for-profit foundation promoting accessible and affordable infertility services in developing countries [71]. The Walking Egg collaborates with the European Society of Human

Reproduction and Embryology and the WHO to make infertility care an integral part of reproductive health care in low-income settings through innovation and research, advocacy and networking, training and capacity building, and service delivery [72].

Affordable Infertility Care

To make infertility care accessible to as many people as possible, it is suggested that services for basic infertility investigations and simple forms of infertility treatment, such as ovulation induction and artificial insemination, might be integrated into existing reproductive health settings [61]. Reduction of costs is also considered a fundamental prerequisite for implementing ARTs in resource-poor countries.

Sallam [66] proposed a model with three levels of assistance:

- A basic infertility clinic offering diagnostic tests and simple forms of infertility treatment
- An advanced clinic where in vitro fertilisation (the simplest procedure) and more advanced diagnostic procedures are available
- A tertiary-level infertility clinic offering specialised assisted reproduction and surgical procedures

Depending on the level of service, funding options include public–private partnership models and partnerships between the World Bank and government, donor agencies, professional societies and the WHO [66].

Standardised investigation of the couple at minimal cost enhances the likelihood of infertile couples seeking assistance. The one-stop diagnostic approach has been proposed, as it includes the responsibility for diagnosis and immediate management policy [71]. The consequences of the results for the management of the couple have to be discussed on the same day.

An accurate history of the couple's personal and medical details, together with a simple light microscopy semen analysis, identifies the majority of infertility problems related to ovulatory dysfunction and male subfertility. As tubal obstruction associated with previous pelvic infections is the greatest cause of infertility in many regions, hysterosalpingography and/or hysterosalpingo-contrast sonography are simple and accessible techniques for detecting this problem without major costs [50]. Office hysteroscopy and diagnostic laparoscopy have also undergone simplification over the years, but are still to be considered second and third-line procedures among infertility investigation techniques.

The diffusion of ARTs in developing countries also requires the adaptation of infertility treatment protocols to low-resource settings. The development of ARTs associated with low costs and a very low complication rate is mandatory if governments are to be convinced to fund infertility clinics. In response, simplified protocols have been developed.

Preliminary awareness of fertility principles by the patients and staff working in the infertility clinics is important within a treatment programme and has been shown to be effective. This awareness includes the importance of timing intercourse to different cervical secretions and the harm caused by smoking and alcohol [6].

Simplicity, safety and cost make clomiphene citrate the first-line treatment for inducing ovulation, provided that tubal patency has been documented, in association with timed intercourse or intra-uterine insemination (IUI).

Gonadotropins represent a second-line agent for inducing ovulation, and their use must be adopted by well-trained and experienced staff, to monitor cycles so as to avoid ovarian hyperstimulation syndrome (OHSS) and to reduce the risk of multiple pregnancies, both complications with devastating consequences in low-resource countries.

In vitro fertilisation represents the logical treatment for tubal infertility and a second-line treatment for infertility. However, the establishment of high-technology assisted reproduction programs in low-resource countries is not only extremely difficult, but also controversial because of the limited healthcare budgets. Simplified protocols have been developed over the years to overcome this obstacle. The use of less potent and cheaper drugs to stimulate oocyte development, minimal monitoring, simplified culture systems and less technologically advanced equipment [73–77] have been proposed as possible methods that may drastically reduce the per-treatment cycle cost, maintaining acceptable live birth rates [73]. Low-cost treatment models through the use of minimal ovarian stimulation and single-embryo transfer would also theoretically eliminate the risk of OHSS and multiple births [76].

Assisted Reproductive Technologies and HIV in Low-Income Countries

A large body of evidence suggests that reproductive technologies can help HIV-affected couples to conceive safely with a minimal risk of HIV transmission to their partner and baby [16]. However, the majority of those affected by HIV live in low-income countries, where such technologies are neither geographically nor economically easily accessible, as discussed above [78–80]. At the end of 2013, there were approximately 35.0 (33.1–37.2) million people living with HIV globally, with sub-Saharan Africa representing the most affected region, with 24.7 (23.4–26.2) million people living with HIV. Moreover, sub-Saharan Africa accounts for almost 70 % of the global total of new HIV infections [81].

Individuals with HIV-seropositive status deserve full reproductive rights and it has been widely demonstrated that simply encouraging HIV-affected couples to abstain from procreation may no longer be a realistic strategy, particularly in communities and cultures where the importance of having children is emphasised [82]. In the absence of counselling that recognises the desire and importance of having children, couples may deliberately take on the risks of transmission to have children, engaging in unprotected intercourse.

In this context, an increasingly crucial issue is the introduction of harm reduction and safer conception methods for people with HIV infection in settings where ART cannot be easily obtained. This is particularly urgent, considering that many countries have recently shown a decline in AIDS-related deaths, but continue to have a high prevalence of HIV infection, largely because of the increased longevity associated with antiretroviral therapy [83].

Most international research on safer conception interventions has been based on settings from industrialised-world contexts and has concentrated on options for couples in which the male partner is infected with HIV and the female partner is not, therefore focusing on "high-technology" methods such as sperm-washing with IUI or in vitro fertilisation/intracytoplasmic sperm injection in laboratory settings.

However, these interventions are not feasible on a widespread basis in resource-constrained settings. Furthermore, in low-income countries, such as in sub-Saharan Africa, most couples are serodiscordant for HIV female positivity, which is different from developed countries, where more men than women are seropositive. As a result, there is a considerable amount of data on the efficacy of sperm-washing, but limited data on timed, unprotected sex, and few data on vaginal insemination [78, 84].

In resource-limited settings, before any safer conception intervention, couples should be counselled and screened in line with the recommendations regarding viral load, CD4+ cell count and sexually transmitted infections. The counsellor should emphasise the need for a close adherence to antiretrovirals to attain an undetectable viral load in the infected partner [85]. Moreover, if the woman is infected, her ART regimen must exclude teratogenic antiretrovirals. Fertility screening is also advisable, if feasible, considering the high prevalence of infertility problems in people with HIV infection [78].

The most feasible method in low-income countries for HIV-serodiscordant couples in which the woman is HIV-seropositive seems to be vaginal self-insemination with sperm from the uninfected male partner, timed to the woman's fertile period [78]. This intervention involves the couple either having intercourse with a condom and then drawing out the semen into a needleless syringe and inserting it as high as possible into the vagina, or the male partner ejaculating into a container and the semen being drawn up in a similar manner. A recent study conducted in Kenya recruited 33 HIV-serodiscordant couples and health-care providers. The authors found that educating and counselling HIV-serodiscordant couples on vaginal insemination could make it an acceptable and feasible safer conception method when associated with frequent communication and home visits by health-care providers [84].

The routine use of vaginal self-insemination as a safe method of conception in HIV-discordant couples for female positivity is of significant public health importance because it is expected to reduce the likelihood of riskier sexual practices (the inconsistent use of male condoms) for childbearing and decrease the incidence of HIV in low-income countries. Systematic research is needed to establish pregnancy rates and outcomes.

For couples in which the man or both partners are positive, the only feasible option is careful, informed natural conception [85]. Timed, limited, unprotected sex for HIV-seroconcordant couples should form part of a harm-reduction strategy to reduce exposure to HIV when planning conception in resource-limited settings.

With regard to HIV-serodiscordant couples with male infection, the use of periconception pre-exposure prophylaxis (PrEP) for the seronegative female partner during timed and limited intercourse is an important method of safer conception. A recent study found strong evidence of the cost-effectiveness of PrEP in South African women, with a reduced mean lifetime risk of HIV from 40 to 27 % [86].

In conclusion, permitting HIV-affected couples safer childbearing is crucial in decreasing both mother-to-child HIV transmission and the infection of seronegative partners.

Further research is needed to establish the awareness, understanding and acceptability of low-technology, safer conception strategies among people with HIV infection.

Conclusion

In developing countries infertility represents a significant problem, and women bear the major burden of this devastating social, medical and economic condition. Developing countries are also afflicted by high rates of HIV infection, with the majority of those affected by HIV living in countries where reproductive technologies for safer conception are not easily accessible.

The diffusion of affordable, effective and safe ARTs in this setting is possible and should be implemented to assist infertile couples and to permit HIV-affected couples safer childbearing, decreasing both vertical and horizontal HIV transmission.

References

1. Cui W. Mother or nothing: the agony of infertility. Bull World Health Organ. 2010;88:881–2. doi:10.2471/BLT.10.011210.
2. ESHRE Task Force on Ethics and Law. Providing infertility treatment in resource-poor countries. Hum Reprod. 2009;24(5):1008–11.
3. Mascarenhas MN, Flaxman SR, Boerma T, Vanderpoel S, Stevens GA. National, regional, and global trends in infertility prevalence since 1990: a systematic analysis of 277 health surveys. PLoS Med. 2012;9(12):e1001356. doi:10.1371/journal.pmed.1001356.
4. Boivin J, Bunting L, Collins JA, Nygren KG. International estimates of infertility prevalence and treatment-seeking: potential need and demand for infertility medical care. Hum Reprod. 2007;22:1506–12. doi:10.1093/humrep/dem046.
5. Rutstein SO, Shah IH. Infecundity, infertility, and childlessness in developing countries. Calverton: ORC Macro; 2004. 57 p.
6. Sharma S, Mittal S, Aggarwal P. Management of infertility in low resource countries. BJOG. 2009;116 Suppl 1:77–83.
7. Cates W, Farley TMM, Row PJ. Worldwide patterns of infertility: is Africa different? Lancet. 1985;2:596–8.
8. World Health Organization. Infections, pregnancies and infertility: perspectives on prevention. Fertil Steril. 1987;47:944–9.
9. Aboulghair MA. The importance of fertility treatment in the developing world. BJOG. 2005;112:1174–6.
10. Ericksen K, Brunette T. Patterns and predictors of infertility among African women: a cross-national survey of twenty-seven nations. Soc Sci Med. 1996;42:209–20.
11. Sciarra JJ. Infertility: a global perspective. The role of pelvic infection. ORGYN. 1994;3:12–5.
12. Ombelet W, Cooke I, Dyer S, Serour G, Devroey P. Infertility and the provision of infertility medical services in developing countries. Hum Reprod Update. 2008;14(6):605–21.
13. Adeniji RA, Olayemi O, Okunlola MA, Aimakhu CO. Pattern of semen analysis of male partners of infertile couples at the University College Hospital, Ibadan. West Afr J Med. 2003;22:243–5.
14. Ikechebelu JI, Adinma JI, Orie EF, Ikegwuonu SO. High prevalence of male infertility in southeastern Nigeria. J Obstet Gynaecol. 2003;23:657–9.
15. Sciarra JJ. Sexually transmitted diseases: global importance. Int J Gynaecol Obstet. 1997;58:107–19.

16. Savasi V, Mandia L, Laoreti A, Cetin I. Reproductive assistance in HIV serodiscordant couples. Hum Reprod Update. 2013;19(2):136–50.

17. Gilling-Smith C, Nicopoullos JD, Semprini AE, Frodsham LC. HIV and reproductive care—a review of current practice. BJOG. 2006;113:869–78.

18. Nabaitu J, Bachengana C, Seeley J. Marital instability in a rural population in south-west Uganda: implications for the spread of HIV-1 infection. Africa (Lond). 1994;64:243–51.

19. Parikh FR, Nadkarni SG, Kumat SA, Naik N, Soonawala SB, Parikh RM. Genital tuberculosis—a major pelvic factor causing infertility in Indian women. Fertil Steril. 1997;67:497–500.

20. Shaheen R, Subhan F, Tahir F. Epidemiology of genital tuberculosis in infertile population. J Pak Med Assoc. 2006;56:306–9.

21. Sharma JB, Roy KK, Pushparaj M, Gupta N, Jain SK, Malhotra N, et al. Genital tuberculosis: an important cause of Asherman's syndrome in India. Arch Gynecol Obstet. 2008;277:33–41.

22. Singh N, Sumana G, Mittal S. Genital tuberculosis: a leading cause of infertility in women seeking assisted conception in north India. Arch Gynecol Obstet. 2008;278:325–7.

23. Grimes DA, Benton J, Singh S, Romero M, Ganatra B, Okonofua FE, et al. Unsafe abortion: the preventable pandemic. Lancet. 2006;238:1908–19.

24. Ganatra B, Tunçalp O, Johnston HB, Johnson Jr BR, Gülmezoglu AM, Temmerman M. From concept to measurement: operationalizing WHO's definition of unsafe abortion. Bull World Health Organ. 2014;92:155. http://dx.doi.org/10.2471/BLT.14.136333.

25. WHO. Unsafe abortion: global and regional estimates of the incidence of unsafe abortion and associated mortality in 2008. 6th ed. Geneva: World Health Organization; 2011.

26. Stanton C, Blanc AK, Croft T, Choi Y. Skilled care at birth in the developing world: progress to date and strategies expanding coverage. J Biosoc Sci. 2007;39:109–20.

27. WHO. Female genital mutilation. Fact sheet No. 241. http://www.who.int/entity/mediacentre/factsheets/fs241/en/index.html (2014).

28. Yoder PS, Khan S. Numbers of women circumcised in Africa: the production of a total. Calverton: Macro International; 2007.

29. Yoder PS, Abderrahim N, Zhuzhuni A. Female genital cutting in the Demographic and Health Surveys: a critical and comparative analysis. Calverton: Macro International; 2004.

30. Obermeyer CM. The consequences of female circumcision for health and sexuality: an update on the evidence. Cult Health Sex. 2005;7:443–61.

31. Dickens BM, Cook RJ. Reproductive health and public health ethics. Int J Gynaecol Obstet. 2007;99:75–9.
32. Bhutta ZA, Salam RA, Das JK. Meeting the challenges of micronutrient malnutrition in the developing world. Br Med Bull. 2013;106:7–17.
33. Cetin I, Berti C, Calabrese S. Role of micronutrients in the periconceptional period. Hum Reprod Update. 2010;16(1):80–95.
34. World Health Organization. World health report, 2000. Geneva: World Health Organization; 2000.
35. Smith K, Corvalán C, Kjellstrom T. How much global ill health is attributable to environmental factors? Epidemiology. 1999;10(5):573–84.
36. WHO. Environment and health in developing countries. http://www. who.int/heli/risks/ehindevcoun/en/. Accessed Sept 2014.
37. Boivin J, Griffiths E, Venetis CA. Emotional distress in infertile women and failure of assisted reproductive technologies: meta-analysis of prospective psychosocial studies. BMJ. 2011;342:d223.
38. Fisher J, Hammarberg K. Psychological and social aspects of infertility in men: an overview of the evidence and implications for psychologically informed clinical care and future research. Asian J Androl. 2012;14:121–9.
39. Dhont N, Temmerman M, van de Wijgert J. Clinical, epidemiological and socio-cultural aspects of infertility in resource-poor settings. Evidence from Rwanda. Facts Views Vis Obgyn. 2011;3(2):77–88.
40. Dyer SJ, Abrahams N, Mokoena NE, van der Spuy ZM. "You are a man because you have children": experiences, reproductive health knowledge and treatment-seeking behaviour among men suffering from couple infertility in South Africa. Hum Reprod. 2004;19:960–7.
41. Dyer SJ, Abrahams N, Mokoena NE, Lombard CJ, van der Spuy ZM. Psychological distress among women suffering from couple infertility in South Africa: a quantitative assessment. Hum Reprod. 2005;20:1938–43.
42. Wiersema NJ, Drukker AJ, Dung MBT, Nhu GH, Nhu NT, Lambalk B. Consequences of infertility in developing countries: results of a questionnaire and interview survey in the south of Vietnam. J Transl Med. 2006;4:54–61.
43. Araoye MO. Epidemiology of infertility: social problems of the infertile couples. West Afr J Med. 2003;22:190–6.
44. Daar AS, Merali Z. Infertility and social suffering: the case of ART in developing countries. In: Vayena E, Rowe PJ, Griffin PD, editors. Current practices and controversies in assisted reproduction. Geneva: World Health Organization; 2002. p. 15–21.

45. Dyer S. The value of children in African countries—insights from studies on infertility. J Psychosom Obstet Gynaecol. 2007;28:69–77.
46. Fledderjohann JJ. 'Zero is not good for me': implications of infertility in Ghana. Hum Reprod. 2012;27:1383–90.
47. Obeisat S, Gharaibeh MK, Oweis A, Gharaibeh H. Adversities of being infertile: the experience of Jordanian women. Fertil Steril. 2012;98:444–9.
48. Papreen N, Sharma A, Sabin K, Begum L, Ahsan SK, Baqui AH. Living with infertility: experiences among urban slum populations in Bangladesh. Reprod Health Matters. 2000;8:33–44.
49. Van Balen F, Inhorn MC. Introduction interpreting infertility: a view from the social sciences. In: Inhorn MC, van Balen F, editors. Infertility around the globe: new thinking on childlessness, gender, reproductive technologies. Berkeley: University of California Press; 2002.
50. Hammarberg K, Kirkman M. Infertility in resource-constrained settings: moving towards amelioration. Reprod Biomed Online. 2013;26(2):189–95.
51. Schenker JG. Assisted reproductive practice: religious perspectives. Reprod Biomed Online. 2005;10(3):310–9.
52. Handwerker L. Social and ethical implications of in vitro fertilization in contemporary China. Camb Q Healthc Ethics. 1995;4:355–63.
53. Qiu RZ. Sociocultural dimensions of infertility and assisted reproduction in the Far East. In: Vayena E, Rowe PJ, Griffin PD, editors. Current practices and controversies in assisted reproduction. Geneva: World Health Organization; 2002. p. 75–8.
54. Macklin R. Reproductive technologies in developing countries. Bioethics. 1995;9:276–81.
55. Daar AS, Merali Z. Infertility and social suffering: the case of ART in developing countries. In: Vayena E, Rowe P, David Griffin P, editors. Current practices and controversies in assisted reproduction "medical, ethical and social aspects of assisted reproduction". Geneva: WHO; 2004. p. 15–21.
56. Tangwa GB. ART and African sociocultural practices: worldview, belief and value systems with particular reference to francophone Africa. In: Vayena E, Rowe PJ, Griffin PD, editors. Current practices and controversies in assisted reproduction. Geneva: World Health Organization; 2002. p. 55–9.
57. WHO Department of Reproductive Health and Research. Accelerating progress towards the attainment of international reproductive health goals and framework for implementing the WHO global reproductive health strategy. Geneva: WHO Department of Reproductive Health and Research; 2006.

58. Indian Council of Medical Research. Need and feasibility of providing assisted technologies for infertility management in resource-poor settings. ICMR Bull. 2000;3:6–7. www.icmr.nic.in.

59. Gerrits T. Biomedical infertility care in low resource countries: barriers and access. Facts Views Vis OBGYN Monogr. 2012:1–6.

60. Inhorn MC. Global infertility and the globalization of new reproductive technologies: illustration from Egypt. Soc Sci Med. 2003;56:1837–51.

61. Ombelet W. Reproductive healthcare systems should include accessible infertility diagnosis and treatment: an important challenge for resource-poor countries. Int J Gynaecol Obstet. 2009;106:168–71.

62. Vayena E, Peterson HB, Adamson D, Nygren K. Assisted reproductive technologies in developing countries: are we caring yet? Fertil Steril. 2009;92:413–6.

63. Potts D, Marks S. Fertility in Southern Africa: the quiet revolution. J South Afr Stud. 2001;27:189–205.

64. United Nations General Assembly. The Universal Declaration of Human Rights (UDHR). www.un.org/en/documents/udhr/ (1948).

65. United Nations International Conference on Population and Development, Cairo. www.un.org/popin/icpd2.htm (1994).

66. Sallam H. Infertility in developing countries: funding the project. ESHRE Monogr. 2008;1:97–101.

67. United Nations Millennium Development Goals. http://www.un.org/millenniumgoals.

68. Fathalla MF, Sinding SW, Rosenfield A, Fathalla MM. Sexual and reproductive health for all: a call for action. Lancet. 2006;368:2095–100.

69. Vayena E, Rowe PJ, Griffin PD. Current practices and controversies in assisted reproduction. Report of a meeting. Geneva: World Health Organization; 2002.

70. ESHRE. http://www.eshre.eu/Specialty-groups/Task-Forces/Task-Force-Developing-Countries-and-Infertility.

71. Ombelet W. Is global access to infertility care realistic? The Walking Egg Project. Reprod Biomed Online. 2014;28:267–72.

72. Ombelet W, van Balen F. Future perspectives. Facts Views Vis OBGYN Monogr. 2012:87–90.

73. Aleyamma TK, Kamath MS, Muthukumar K, Mangalaraj AM, George K. Affordable ART: a different perspective. Hum Reprod. 2011;26:3312–8.

74. Cooke ID, Gianaroli L, Hovatta O, Trounson A. Affordable ART in the Third World: difficulties to overcome. ESHRE Monogr. 2008;1:93–6.

75. Hovatta O, Cooke ID. Cost-effective approaches to in vitro fertilization: means to improve access. Int J Gynaecol Obstet. 2006; 94:287–92.
76. Ombelet W, Campo R. Affordable IVF for developing countries. Reprod Biomed Online. 2007;15:257–65.
77. Van Blerkom J, Ombelet W, Klerkx E, Janssen M, Dhont N, Nargund G, Campo R. First births with a simplified culture system for clinical IVF and ET. Reprod Biomed Online. 2013;28:310–20.
78. Chadwick RJ, Mantell JE, Moodley J, Harries J, Zweigenthal V, Cooper D. Safer conception interventions for HIV-affected couples: implications for resource-constrained settings. Top Antivir Med. 2011;19(4):148–55.
79. Frodsham LC, Boag F, Barton S, Gilling-Smith C. Human immunodeficiency virus infection and fertility care in the United Kingdom: demand and supply. Fertil Steril. 2006;85(2):285–9.
80. Stanitis JA, Grow DR, Wiczyk H. Fertility services for human immunodeficiency virus-positive patients: provider policy, practice, and perspectives. Fertil Steril. 2008;89(5):1154–8.
81. WHO. HIV/AIDS. Fact sheet N°360. Updated Jul 2014; 2014.
82. Erhabor O, Akani CI, Eyindah CE. Reproductive health options among HIV-infected persons in the low-income Niger Delta of Nigeria. HIV AIDS. 2012;4:29–35.
83. Myer L, Carter RJ, Katyal M, Toro P, El-Sadr WM, Abrams EJ. Impact of antiretroviral therapy on incidence of pregnancy among HIV-infected women in Sub-Saharan Africa: a cohort study. PLoS Med. 2010;7(2):e1000229.
84. Mmeje O, van der Poel S, Workneh M, Njoroge B, Bukusi E, Cohen CR. Achieving pregnancy safely: perspectives on timed vaginal insemination among HIV-serodiscordant couples and health-care providers in Kisumu, Kenya. AIDS Care. 2015;27(1):10–6. Epub 2014 Aug 8.
85. Matthews LT, Mukherjee JS. Strategies for harm reduction among HIV-affected couples who want to conceive. AIDS Behav. 2009;13 Suppl 1:5–11.
86. Walensky RP, Park JE, Wood R, Freedberg KA, Scott CA, Bekker LG, Losina E, Mayer KH, Seage III GR, Paltiel AD. The cost-effectiveness of pre-exposure prophylaxis for HIV infection in South African women. Clin Infect Dis. 2012;54(10):1504–13.

Index

© Springer International Publishing Switzerland 2016
A. Borini, V. Savasi (eds.), *Assisted Reproductive Technologies and Infectious Diseases*,
DOI 10.1007/978-3-319-30112-9